"What happens when sperm meets egg, and dude becomes dad-to-be? Life as you know it changes forever—and, you're surprised to find, you wouldn't have it any other way. *From Dude to Dad* tells it like it is, and like it will be, with humor, empathy, insight, and practical relatable advice on everything from easing your partner's queasiness to handling hormones (hers and yours), sex and romance to birth plans and car seats."

—Heidi Murkoff, *What to Expect When You're Expecting*

"As a father of three and someone who has dedicated my life to healthy families, there is a moment of awakening (and panic!) that happens from the moment you find out you're expecting. From practical information to sensitive considerations and humor, this book has it all for new dads!"

—Christopher Gavigan, founder of the Honest Company/ Honest.com

"If you're a dude going to be a dad, this book will make you laugh all the way to fatherhood!"

—Adam Cohen, DaDaRocks.com

FROM DUDE TO DAD

THE DIAPER DUDE
GUIDE TO PREGNANCY

Chris Pegula with Frank Meyer

A PERIGEE BOOK

A PERIGEE BOOK
Published by the Penguin Group
Penguin Group (USA) LLC
375 Hudson Street, New York, New York 10014

USA • Canada • UK • Ireland • Australia • New Zealand • India • South Africa • China

penguin.com

A Penguin Random House Company

FROM DUDE TO DAD

ISBN: 978-0-399-16626-6

An application to register this book for cataloging has been
submitted to the Library of Congress.

First edition: May 2014

PRINTED IN THE UNITED STATES OF AMERICA

10 9 8 7 6 5 4 3 2 1

Text design by Laura K. Corless

Neither the publisher nor the author is engaged in rendering professional advice or services to
the individual reader. The ideas, procedures, and suggestions contained in this book are not
intended as a substitute for consulting with your physician. All matters regarding your health
require medical supervision. Neither the author nor the publisher shall be liable or responsible
for any loss or damage allegedly arising from any information or suggestion in this book.

While the author has made every effort to provide accurate telephone numbers,
Internet addresses, and other contact information at the time of publication, neither the
publisher nor the author assumes any responsibility for errors, or for changes that occur
after publication. Further, the publisher does not have any control over and does not
assume any responsibility for author or third-party websites or their content.

Most Perigee books are available at special quantity discounts for bulk purchases for sales
promotions, premiums, fund-raising, or educational use. Special books, or book excerpts, can
also be created to fit specific needs. For details, write: Special.Markets@us.penguingroup.com.

To Meredith, my soul mate, best friend, and muse.
I love you.

And Dad.
Thank you for being an example I hope to be able to live up to.
I love you.

Contents

Chapter 5: Life with Baby 115

Chapter 6: Happy and Healthy Parenting 139

How We Got Here

I wake up to the sound of crying. Barely coherent, my brain still asleep, I glance at the clock and make out the time. It's 5 a.m. Crap.

I roll over to find my wife gone. In a slow-motion panic, I drag my body out of bed. As I struggle to open my eyes, which have been sealed shut by sleep, I am following the sounds of sobbing toward the bathroom when I hear something drop to the floor. Uh-oh: Has she received some late night bad news? Did somebody die? As I scurry toward the light, I catch a glimpse through a crack in the door of my wife holding what looks like a thermometer. Double crap.

Just as I psych myself up for an early morning CVS run for meds or cough syrup or whatever it is she needs, I hear the words. "We're pregnant!"

THUMP! It hits like a rock. All the color drains from my face and tears roll down my cheeks. Tears of joy or fear, I'm not sure, but it is the moment I've been waiting for my whole life. It's really happening. What do I know about parenting? Sometimes I forget to feed the dog. What if I forget to feed the kid!

"Are you sure?" I ask.

"I took the test three times," she replies through the biggest smile I have ever seen in my life. As I gaze at this woman who will soon be raising our children and providing our family with wisdom and guidance, my life flashes across my brain. My first kiss with Carrie Gombetti playing spin the bottle in the garage at her birthday party. Sister Natalie, my high school Sex Ed teacher, who taught me that I'd go straight to hell with no parole if I even thought about doing IT (which I was okay with as long as I got to touch some boobs at some point in my life). Scoring for the first time at a Friday night football game with Cindy Borovsky (and I'm not talking about a field goal!). My first car. My first job. Sex. College. Meeting my wife. Proposing to her on one knee. Sex. Our wedding. Even better, our wedding night. The honeymoon. More sex.

So what's going to happen now? Will I ever be able to hang with the guys again? Am I allowed to have fun once I'm a dad? What if we suck at this parenting game? Do they take your kids away? How will my wife's body change? Will we ever have sex again?

Any of this sound familiar?

Dude, relax.

If you're anything like me (and according to many women we're all exactly the same), all of this stuff crossed your mind when you found out you were going to be a dad. It's normal.

Don't worry. You're going to be fine. But it wouldn't hurt to get a few pointers, a road map if you will, as to what lies ahead.

That is what this book is for.

One of the reasons I wrote this book was because when my wife got pregnant there wasn't much on the shelves for men explaining what to do when she's expecting. Oh, there were plenty of books for women about the ins and outs of childbirth, but the options for dads were slim. Either they were these clinical, scientific tomes that read like homework, or they were nudge-nudge wink-wink sarcastic in tone. Lots of dick jokes and boob humor. Not really my style and definitely nothing my wife would ever buy me. So I thought maybe it was time for something that tells dads what to do when their partner is pregnant in an honest, factual, fun way; a book that takes you step-by-step through all three trimesters, plus the prep to get there and the aftermath. It's Pregnancy 101 from the dude's point of view.

Throughout this book, you'll learn what you need to know when she gets pregnant, how to handle the big news, how early you can start telling folks, and which doctor appointments are important for you to attend. You'll learn also how you can help your partner, how you can maintain a strong relationship with your significant other while helping her through pregnancy. And yes, we will discuss your sex life for the next nine months. Allow me to cut right to the chase on that one: you'll still have one.

Dude, don't worry, life ain't over.

As your kids grow up, being a dad is an ever-changing role, but probably the most baffling time is those first nine months when your wife or partner is carrying the child. So much information comes flying at you. And the idea that you two will become three is exciting . . . but terrifying. Again, don't worry: I went through this stuff three times and even started my own business based on what I learned from being a dad. In fact, it might help to know how I started that business, so you know where I'm coming from and why I strongly believe you can maintain your own identity while still being a dad. Allow me to give you a little history lesson . . .

The Diaper Dude Philosophy

One day about a decade ago, my very pregnant wife Meredith came home from shopping armed with a dozen flowery diaper bags. I took one look at them and said, "Is one of these supposed to be for me?" She said I could take my pick. My eyes glazed over looking at one girly pink sack after the other before I muttered, "There's no way in hell I can walk around with that strapped to my side. Can't you find one that is more . . . er, manly?" She assured me they didn't make diaper bags for men and to just to pick one and get over it.

"Hell, I could make one better than these things," I boasted. She laughed.

At the time I was an actor and a stay-at-home dad with my own dog walking business. Since I really wanted something that reflected my style and there was nothing out there, I decided to start my own company. Problem was, I had no retail or manufacturing experience, no idea how to even begin such an endeavor, and had never run a large business before. But it seemed like there was a need for products for fathers, and I decided to go for it. I launched Diaper Dude a little over ten years ago on Father's Day, and things took off from there.

What started off as a simple concept, to make a cool diaper bag for myself, eventually turned into my mission statement: *You do not have to lose who you are when you become a dad.*

There's this idea that once you become a parent, your life is over and you must totally transform yourself to fit the role of a dad. Many guys think, "Oh shit, I'm stuck with the family, I can't be spontaneous or travel anymore, none of my friends will think I'm still cool with a kid around . . ." and so on.

Those fears were there for me too until I realized that having kids was actually an amazing new chapter in my life, and that I was gaining incredible life experiences that far outweighed those from my life as a bachelor. Sure, life got a little more complex, but being a father gave me a whole new outlook on life. The truth is, you can still be who you are after you become a parent; you simply gain a bigger world in which to be yourself. And it's not all about YOU anymore. Your universe expands to include your child and the lady in your life.

And remember, her life is changing too. It's often difficult for men to feel connected to the experience their wife or partner is going through. She has a baby growing inside of her, her body is changing, and she is showing all these strange symptoms you barely understand (weight gain, cravings, mood swings). We're left to the side scratching our heads, thinking, "Where do I fit in? How do I handle all of this?"

I hope this book can show you that you count too: you have just as important a role to play—this is your baby too! Hey, it takes two to tango . . . and two to make a baby. But you've figured that out by now, right? (Please say yes . . .)

CHAPTER

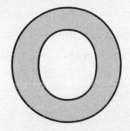

Before the Countdown Begins

Meredith and I were both twenty-seven when she got pregnant with our first child. She has lupus, an autoimmune disease, and we knew our pregnancy would most likely be considered high risk. But Meredith's sister was pregnant with her second child, my siblings had begun having children, and we had a few friends who were pregnant with their first child, so we felt like the time was right. Actually, my feeling is that you are never going to be totally prepared, and part of the experience is learning as you go along, so you might as well jump!

Our first doctor didn't provide us with the experience we hoped for, medically or emotionally. We assumed he would look at Meredith's disease in relation to her pregnancy and give us insight into what we might have in store for us over the next nine months in a straightforward yet sensitive manner.

Seems reasonable, right? This was hardly the case. In our only appointment with this man, he began to speak in a stream-of-consciousness manner on the many negative realities of having lupus and children. Essentially, this man, without educating himself on my wife's individual case, made a broad judgment that our pregnancy would most likely be riddled with complications resulting in the baby being stillborn. My wife and I left his office in tears and feeling hopeless. Fortunately we did not let that experience dictate our future.

We found another doctor and got a second opinion. Thankfully, the second doctor felt confident that there was no reason we couldn't have a healthy baby and that we should start trying whenever we were ready (which was immediately). As it turned out, a high-risk doctor wasn't even needed, for any of my wife's three pregnancies. (The moral of the story? Don't settle on one opinion. Especially not the first one you hear. Explore your options and get a second, even third, opinion if necessary.)

Once we got the green light, we were eager to begin. I was psyched I didn't need to wear a condom anymore. However, we soon learned that there is a science behind making babies. It's not all fun and games. Some people have it easier than others. I was prepared to take as long as we needed to hit a home run, if you will. My wife, on the other hand, was militant about it being sooner than later, for fear of striking out.

After we were unsuccessful the first month, Meredith learned about kits that help women in determining the exact time of ovulation so they can try during their most fertile period, thereby increasing chances of success. The second month was our first experience with the ovulation kit, but it took another month before we got it right. In our case, the ol' saying "third time's a charm" was true, because the forces of nature finally collided and formed our little dude, now known as Kai.

Little did I know the journey that I was about to embark on . . .

Thinking back, I was in no way prepared to be a father, emotionally or financially. I was young, in love, and enthusiastic, but did not have a career in place, a steady income or any idea of what it meant to be a father (least of all a father of three, like I am now). But I soon found out that, with the help of my wife, I could rise to the challenge and become a terrific dad—if I do say so myself—and all it took was some motivation, education, and preparation.

PREPPING FOR IMPREGNATING

How the two of you can get prepared to make babies.

Parenting is a lot like marathon training. It's a huge commitment and very exhausting, yet the reward once you cross that finish line is beyond description (I know this being a marathon runner myself). So once you decide to start the baby making process, think of your body like you're an athlete about to train for a marathon.

First, head to your doctor for a checkup. There are all sorts of things she can do to get herself ready for pregnancy, but you too can prep your body for baby making. Think about it. Are you physically ready for this? Be smart and don't rely alone on your manly instinct that you are in killer shape. For instance, no one wants varicose veins. But you *really* don't want them in the scrotum, as they can alter your sperm. Nice visual,

DUDE, TREAT YOUR BODY RIGHT

When you begin the baby making process, your partner may ask that you too start making changes from the very beginning, including eating healthier, quitting smoking, or laying off the bourbon (or at least cutting it in half). As well, *you* should eliminate as many medications from your routine as possible. Yes, YOU. Talk with your physician about your prescription medications, as you may need to discontinue using some and try something new. Why? Medications such as Tagamet (cimetidine), sulfasalazine, and nitrofurantoin, which are used to treat gastrointestinal problems, ulcers, and urinary tract infections, have been known to impact male fertility, negatively affecting both sperm production and count. Yikes!

eh? You might even consider taking it easy on the biking since there have been some suggestions it might be linked to low sperm production, although there is no definitive reason why this is the case. (It may be due to the position, the clothing, or the heat created in that area, but why risk it, right?) Using hot tubs might also become an issue with your sperm production, due to what is referred to as wet heat. Of course, get advice from your physician on these specific topics to be safe. I had no idea at the time that any of that stuff was a concern. Getting into the mind-set of thinking not only of yourself but of your family from this point on will help make the adjustment to being a parent easier.

Understand *you* may be asked to undergo genetic testing for conditions such as cystic fibrosis, Down syndrome, and Tay-Sachs. It was a surprise to me when I learned that being

Eastern European could play a role in specific diseases that we could be vulnerable to if I carried the gene, namely Tay-Sachs. Fortunately, I did not. But I remember how freaked out I was about the waiting period after I took the tests. What-ifs can drive you nuts. Think about how women feel having to endure months of tests—what-ifs, couldas, hopefullys, and so on. My wife is way stronger than me in that department, and I think that's why I felt an extreme desire, obligation even, to assist in any way I could to make this process as enjoyable and memorable for her as possible. Keep in mind, she's the one enduring all the pain, bodily changes, and risk. The least you can do is help her through it, right? At the end of the day, all the testing and prep is for the health of your baby, so if you can go in knowing you are arming yourself with information that will serve you for the better, you may reduce the stress you both feel while waiting for the results down the line.

And while you are in this nerve-wracking phase, don't forget to occasionally go do something you enjoy, that makes you feel good (but for the next nine months, try not to make that a stiff drink!), because along with making sure you're physically fit, you'll also want to maintain a positive mind-set. You can help steer the ship as far as emotions and reactions go. As you're trying to get pregnant, the last thing your lady wants to hear is that you aren't ready or don't think you can do it. And remember: both of you have a fair amount of fear involved, and you only have nine months to get yourself ready emotionally, financially, and beyond.

If at first you don't succeed, do not get frustrated or play the blame game. There are a handful of times in your life when you must rise to the challenge in the sex department. Think back to the first time you ever did it. It was terrifying, but you stepped up to the plate and took a swing! Or the first time you were with a *really* hot girl, the kind so out of your league you actually questioned your own ability to pleasure her without embarrassing yourself. Well, dude, *this* is one of those times. If at first you don't succeed . . . well, you know the rest. Use your powers, your energy, and your sex drive to stay on top of this and keep trying.

Over the years, if there's one thing I have learned about maintaining a sex life, it's to stay passionate. Of course, passion is a relative term; to each his or her own. But whatever it is that makes the two of you hot for each other, do those things! Make your partner want you, make her long for you, and then make her feel good. At the end of the day, even though you are making babies, you are still making love. Taking the time to be in the moment, enjoy each other, and have fun can help to eliminate the stress surrounding what can sometimes feel as much like a scheduled commitment as an act of passion.

Support your partner, be a good listener, and allow her to vent her frustrations during this time. If you are lucky enough to strike it rich the first time out, fantastic. But chances

---

⟶ KEEP COOL

One study cited that sperm counts in five out of eleven men with fertility problems increased by 491 percent after they stopped taking baths or using the hot tub for a few months. Sperm is made optimally at slightly below body temperature, so think about wearing boxer shorts instead of tighty-whities, and don't spend too long in warm baths, as colder conditions improve circulation around the testicles.

> ➤ **DID YOU KNOW?**
>
> Heavy drinking can affect sperm quality and make a successful pregnancy less likely, say experts. Other health-related causes of lower sperm count include steroids, obesity, heavy tobacco smoking, and extreme emotional stress.

are it could take more attempts to hit a home run. It is important for your partner to have a shoulder for *anything*—to lean on or cry on. Your shoulder isn't the only thing she'll need. Listen to her—her hopes and her fears. My wife cried *a lot* the first month, when we were striking out. She thought she would never get pregnant, so this was a very emotional time for her.

Since she is the one actually getting pregnant, she's under much more pressure during this process. Be a real man and be rock solid for your partner. Don't buy into the bullshit stereotypes that men cannot be supportive or expressive when it comes to pregnancy. I can guarantee it's more attractive to a woman to have a man who will listen and support her than someone who thinks pregnancy is a female problem *she* needs to deal with. After all, who are you trying to impress, her or your friends? Don't get sucked into stereotypes. If you can't support her now, how do you expect to do it once your little one arrives?

SHE'S PREGNANT!

She has nine months to prepare for this baby. You have to get your act together . . . NOW!

So the time comes when you discover your boys did the job. How do you react?

Perhaps you didn't plan for this to happen. Hey, it happens to the best of us. But we are all adults here, and if you are having sex without a condom and/or she's not on the pill, then you know you are taking a risk. So don't be so shocked when she comes to you with the news.

And if this wasn't a planned moment in your relationship? I spoke to a friend who openly admitted that his first kid was definitely an accident. Though his initial response was "Shit, really?" He soon followed up with "All right!!! I'm gonna be a dad!" and immediately went into the mode of taking the relationship to the next level by assuming responsibility and openly welcoming the notion of being a parent. Him turning into a solid dad was no accident.

Of course, if you were planning the pregnancy from the

DID YOU KNOW?

Did you know that at the moment of fertilization, your baby's genetic makeup is complete, including its sex? In a mere thirteen weeks, what begins as a single cell becomes a tiny fetus, complete with recognizable human features and all of a baby's internal organs in place.

beginning, then you most likely will feel the three stages of pregnancy reaction among dudes:

1. Relief
2. Excitement
3. Fear
4. Already?

First there is a sense of relief because if you're trying to get your partner pregnant, there is always that fear that it won't happen for whatever reason. You'll have a sperm problem or she'll have an egg problem or something terrible will happen because it always does, and so on.

But that isn't the case this time, and then comes the excitement. Hell yeah! I'm gonna be a dad! Woo hoo!!!! Cigars, champagne, handshakes, hugs and kisses will follow in mass quantities. This is good.

Until it's not. Then there is bone-chilling fear. It dawns on you that YOU are going to be responsible for another life. Not a girlfriend you can break up with or a wife who can take care of herself if you divorce. But a child! YOU of all people. You are a moron! You know this. I am too. We all are! All this sets in for a few minutes but then fades away. We're not morons. We're just men.

Then for a minute—just a minute—you get a little bit bummed out. Not because you don't want to be a father, but because you were having soooo much fun trying to have a baby that you wonder if your sex life will ever be that rowdy and raucous again. I mean, it got crazy there for a while, right? Something about knowing that there was a purpose to the sex, that it truly was lovemaking (literally making something out

of love) made it even more special . . . and hot! But will it ever
be that exciting again? Don't worry, dude. It can be. Trust me.

The reality is that you are having a kid. Whether your pregnancy was planned or crept up unexpectedly, both of you have
a new road ahead of you. In fact, now is a good time to start
thinking of your role for the next nine months. Most of the
work is gonna fall on your partner, so it's important for you to
shoulder some of the weight to make it easier. You can help
make this a wonderful experience you both will never forget.

But when can you start telling other people?

IT'S A CELEBRATION, Y'ALL! . . . OR IS IT?

*Who to tell she's preggers and when at this early stage. Don't
be a social network blabbermouth, dude . . .*

Sharing the good news with my friends and family was one of
my favorite parts of my wife's pregnancy. I can still hear my

---

⟶ IN VITRO

In vitro fertilization is a major treatment for infertility when
other methods of assisted reproductive technology have
failed. It is the process by which an egg is fertilized by sperm
outside the body (the "in vitro" part) by removing ovum (eggs)
from a woman's ovaries and letting the sperm fertilize one of
them in a laboratory test tube. The fertilized egg (aka the zy-
gote) is then transferred to the woman's uterus. Hence the
term "test tube baby."

mom's high-pitched "OOOOOOH!" ringing in my ears. Since I was the fifth of six kids, I think it really hit home for her because I was one of the babies of the clan. Now I was having a baby!

Meredith and I talked a lot about whether we would share our pregnancy news immediately or wait until the first trimester had passed. But my wife knows that I suck at keeping secrets, and she was so overjoyed that it was almost impossible for her to keep her mouth shut, so we decided to share the news right off the bat. Additionally, since lupus was already a part of our world, we decided it was better to have an army of loved ones to be there if we experienced complications that compromised the pregnancy.

Many women, however, understandably fear leaking the news too soon (usually during the first trimester) in case there are complications that lead to a miscarriage. So many couples may decide together not to tell anyone. But how do you keep *that* quiet? You want to celebrate but you can't yet. And when you do tell people, it doesn't always come out right. For instance, when my wife told her folks, she just casually slipped the word "grandparents" into a normal conversation and waited until they went, "Wait, what did you say?!?" Priceless.

If you simply must share the news, consider mutually agreeing upon a few select confidants, a first wave of confidants if you will. For instance, we told our parents and best friends (who became the godparents) first, and then a few days later our siblings. After the first trimester we let the rest of the world in on the good news (more on that later). A friend of mine once told me that a good rule for telling people about a pregnancy was that you tell the exact same group of people you would also tell if there was a miscarriage: the people who are your support system. Decide together who gets included in that first round of baby news and who gets to be in the next wave.

WHAT'S UP, DOC?

Do I have to go? And if so, which appointments do I need to attend and which can I skip?

Dude, I hate to break it to ya, but you need to go to many, if not all, of your partner's doctor's appointments during her pregnancy. Don't forget that she is the one who will soon be pushing a butterball out of her lady parts, so it's the least you can do. Seriously, be there for your partner. Your support will often be just what she needs. And when it's not needed, stay out of the way.

Throughout our marriage we have had many a relationship with my wife's doctors. Talk about having a threesome! The truth is, having an autoimmune disease can demand consistent medical attention. I couldn't imagine my wife being alone during her doctor visits, so it was a no-brainer when it came to her pregnancy. I wanted to be there for any and all possible news, good or bad.

Our first sonogram experience was one neither one of us will ever forget. During the exam the doctor showed us a sonogram of our growing baby and confirmed the due date. For the first time, we got to see the baby's image on the screen. Of course, it was so tiny and globby at this point that I was impressed the doctor could even make out that my wife was pregnant! But trust me, seeing that image of your child for the first

THE CYCLE OF
THE MENSTRUATION CYCLE

Due dates are determined by the first day of your partner's last menstrual period. The menstrual cycle is divided into three phases: First, the body gets ready to ovulate. Then ovulation. Lastly, if that month's egg hasn't been fertilized, menstruation begins. Timing sex with the release of an egg gives you the best chance at conception. The most fertile times of a woman's cycle are a few days before she ovulates and/or the actual day of ovulation. There is only one window of time per month when she can be impregnated, before you need to wait another thirty days or so and try again. Looking at it from that point of view really clues you in as to why it's so much tougher on women when it takes a long time to get pregnant.

time will take your breath away and make the constant doctor visits totally worth it.

There will be many appointments that will mark milestones in her pregnancy, important benchmarks you will need to be there for, such as her first prenatal visit (where you find out the due date) and the ultrasound (see the little critter!). Be there.

This seemingly endless barrage is just a part of the journey, amigo. Go to as many as humanly possible. From hearing the heartbeat for the first time, to discovering the sex of your baby if you choose to, these visits can be a time for you to bond as a couple. These appointments are also among the first times dads get to really feel like a part of the experience. Therefore, these are also good times for you to ask questions.

There will even be moments when your partner will count on you to call her doctor when she is having symptoms that are freaking her out. Sometimes having *you* make the call relieves her anxiety. It's also good for you to put a face to the name of the doctor who will be with you in the delivery room come baby time. The delivery room isn't where you wanna meet for the first time the person who will be staring into your wife's nether regions! Aaawkward.

Look at it this way, what could you possibly have to do that's more important than attending these visits with your partner? Whatever it may be, move it. Prioritize! The earlier you start making adjustments to your life, the easier the transition into parenthood will be.

While there are a variety of appointments she will have with her doctor that are scheduled ahead of time, sometimes something unexpected occurs and you both may want to rush to the emergency room. Often a simple call to her OBGYN can help ease any anxiety you both may be feeling. Let a professional assess whether further medical attention is needed. Not every episode requires a trip to the emergency room, but better safe than sorry. Being overprepared is rarely a bad thing in this new phase of your life . . .

DUDE, YOUR LIFE ISN'T OVER

What she is going through and what the hell you can do about it.

Okay, the big ol' baby bomb has been dropped. She gave you the big news and you are either freaking out or on cloud nine.

You have nine months to prepare for the arrival of your little one. What can you do during that time to help out and get ready for the next phase of your life?

First off, you need to be emotionally prepared. Don't worry, I'm not going to get all spiritual and Dr. Philish on ya. I just mean that there are going to be a lot of changes going on in your household, specifically when it comes to your relationship with your wife, and you should be ready for them. Sometimes that simply means that when she handles things differently or reacts more emotionally than she did in the past, you have to roll with it.

We've all heard of hormones, right? We'll talk more about them later, but hormones are basically chemical messengers that carry a signal from one cell to another. They are like emails traveling throughout the human body system. Those li'l suckers are running rampant in your wife's system right now and making her act differently than before. More extreme. More emotional. It's not unusual for her to burst into tears over things you find to be trivial and hardly worth the drama. It's totally normal, dude.

The reality is that women are tough as hell. They endure nearly a year of emotional and physical changes that we men can never truly relate to. I shudder to think of the pain endured during delivery. Forgive the crude analogy, but imagine pooping a basketball out your backside and you begin to get the picture. So if you can stay sensitive to the changes she is experiencing during this period and take into account that she is not her usual self for a very good reason, your lives will be much easier.

How do you stay sensitive? Well, one way is by being attentive to the physical changes your partner is experiencing. Ask her how she is feeling and what she is feeling. Do a little readin' up on what happens during each of the three trimesters. Offer her some complimentary words to remind her that you are still physically attracted to her. Pregnant women have a certain glow about them that is really attractive. Reminding her that she is still hot will boost her ego and keep you on her good side. And believe you me, you do not want her to go to the dark side. The force is strong there, young Jedi, and will punch you in the gut!

"So what can I do about it?" you demand again. Well, you can make sure your partner is taking care of herself and help her out as much as possible, make sure she gets plenty of sleep at night and that she also takes breaks throughout the day to chill out and relax. Encourage her to regularly get exercise and engage in physical activity (but make sure she doesn't push herself too hard). She's got to eat well, take plenty of naps, yet stay social and active.

Mainly though, you can help her feel good about herself, take away some stress, talk her off the ledge when things get tense, and give massages . . . lots and lots of massages. Being sensitive to her emotions will surely keep you out of trouble.

→ DID YOU KNOW?

About one week after her missed period, her pregnancy will be visible on ultrasound. Sure, it is merely a small fluid collection (called a gestational sac), within the lining of the uterus, that's only about two-tenths of an inch in diameter, but it's your kid, dude!

Many women can feel unattractive and overweight when they are pregnant and after, even when they've lost the weight. So say nice things to make her feel sexy during and after the pregnancy.

Validation is a major key. She won't always want you to fix things or have a solution, but instead just to say, "Wow, I hear what you're saying." There will be times when she will erupt over things that seem just plain ridiculous to you. Do not tell her she is being silly or that whatever she is upset about is not worth her time. This stuff is important to her at that moment. It may pass, it may not, but don't trivialize her emotions. Just take the heat and move on.

There are also times when you will be tempted to engage in battle over things as you did in the pre-pregnancy days. Before you open your mouth, stop, take a deep breath, and think about how important the issue is to you. Is the fact that she misplaced your copy of *Call of Duty* really *that* important to you in the big picture? Or that she gave away the last beer in the fridge to the thirsty neighbor she was chatting with earlier? Normally this stuff might annoy you to death and you'd say something. But knowing that she's more sensitive now and may just not be thinking of you every second of the day like she used to (you know, because of that growing baby in her tummy taking up all her attention), choose your battles a little more carefully.

Of course, that doesn't mean be a wimp. If she did something big like cheat on you or slug down bottles of wine while pregnant, it would certainly be worth saying something.

If you can anchor yourself, stay calm, clear, and open-minded, you will better deflect potential disasters. Listen to her tone, observe her mannerisms, and try to understand why she is upset. Use phrases like "What I am hearing is that you are upset at me for leaving my underwear on the bedroom floor . . . again?" or "I understand you are upset over [fill in your latest screwup here], and I'd like to try and make it up to you." You'd be surprised how often simply acknowledging that you are listening to what she is saying does the trick. Remember, don't try to solve the problem, per se, just listen and say you'll try to do better. We can only try, my man.

I know this may sound like you need to be soft and may even seem emasculating to some of you, but get over it. Imagine being pumped up with gallons and gallons of caffeine, getting the runs for an hour, and then being dehydrated, all in a matter of minutes. Sounds excruciating, right? Now imagine your body experiencing this for nine whole months. *That* is what she is dealing with. And now so are you. Enjoy.

Remember . . .

- Careful how you handle the news with your partner. She needs a teammate.

- Be selective as to who you tell at this early stage and decide together.

- Go to as many doctor appointments with her as possible.

- Be sensitive. She needs your support and understanding.

- Relax. Your life isn't over, dude.

CHAPTER

1

The First Trimester

As you enter the first trimester, this starts to get real. All that stuff you've read about and seen in movies begins to manifest itself in true-life situations. Yes, she probably will get nauseous. Yes, that nausea will soon turn into morning sickness. Her hormones are fluctuating, and she really does have heightened sensitivity. You'll need to be flexible during this time. I quickly learned that Meredith was pretty much MIA during those first three months. Her energy was really depleted, and nausea basically kicked her butt. I still have visions of her in bed and not seeing her face for what seemed like days. You'll most likely encounter similar transitions, so being open to change is beneficial.

What exactly is a trimester? Here's some basics, dude. Your partner's pregnancy is divided into three of 'em. Each is broken down into three months, for a total of nine, hence the "tri" in trimester. She will experience pretty significant changes in each trimester, so it's a good idea to sign up for a pregnancy calendar to see what she is undergoing week by week (we've included a basic one in the back of the book for you too). You'll want to know what is around the corner as much as possible, and it's pretty remarkable to see how quickly your little one develops in the first trimester alone.

"When my wife got pregnant, my schedule went out the window," a close friend of mine recently recollected. "Anything could come up at any time, and it did. I realized if I was going to be a good partner, then I'd better be flexible. Like water. Water fills any new space it comes in contact with. We need to be more like water." A little abstract, but I agree. Think of yourself like water in this regard. Hey, with the amount of coffee and/or beer going in and pee coming out, the analogy is not that far off!

Yet while you want to be flexible, don't forget *your* role here either. We too go to great lengths for our family—not just working hard to provide food, shelter, and entertainment, but providing a shoulder to cry on and a listening ear, and being a beacon of strength and reason during these emotional times.

Make sure you carve out time for yourself too. If you have hobbies, continue to do them. If you love sports, stay active. Part of not losing who you are as you become a father is to hold on to as much of your interests, abilities, personality traits, and quirks as you can. You know, the stuff that attracted her to you in the first place, the stuff that makes you YOU! At the same time, include her in these things as much as possible. If you play ball with the guys every Sunday morning, invite her to come picnic and watch. If you are a movie buff, take her along. Check in with her, plan out fun things to do together, and encourage her to keep up with her hobbies as well.

WHERE ARE WE NOW?

Her condition, what she needs from you, and how her body is feeling.

By the end of the first trimester your baby has formed and is restin' in her tummy. Trippy, eh? And it keeps growing and growing! In fact, at this stage the baby is developing internal organs such as the heart, brain, lungs, and kidneys. Its little baby heart starts to beat and yours will probably skip a beat when you hear it for the first time. (Dude, this is a moment you will never forget, so you definitely want to be there. If you have never openly wept before, be prepared.) Despite not looking pregnant much yet, your partner is gonna start going through morning sickness and exhaustion, and cravings will be kicking in.

Even though she may be feeling lousy, her body is working in high gear. Your developing baby is called an embryo from the moment of conception to the eighth week of pregnancy. After the eighth week and until the moment of birth, your baby is called a fetus. By week five your baby's heart and circulatory system are forming and by week six your baby's face is taking shape. By week eleven that little creature inside is starting to look human. And by the close of the first trimester, your pipsqueak is about the size of a peach!

During the first trimester her body undergoes many changes. Hormonal changes affect almost every organ system and can trigger symptoms as soon as the first few weeks of pregnancy. In addition to her period stopping, changes may include:

- Extreme tiredness
- Tender, swollen breasts; her nipples might also stick out
- Morning sickness
- Cravings or distaste for certain foods
- Mood swings
- Constipation
- Need to pee more often
- Headache
- Heartburn
- Weight gain or loss

Women can start feeling nauseous as early as three weeks after conception. There are some things that she can try to help her get relief from the nausea, such as motion sickness wristbands, ginger tea, popsicles, smoothies, and crackers. But what she will need most of all is you to lean on, figuratively and literally.

You need to make an extra effort not to be a pain in her neck during these months (it's hard, I know, it comes so naturally to us men). Late nights with the guys and double shifts at work are probably not a wise decision for a while. Adjust your schedule so you can be around for her as much as she needs. It can get pretty unnerving to see your partner feel so shitty for so long. That's why being part of her doctor visits can arm

> ⟶ **DAD NIGHT OUT**
>
> While I highly advise being flexible about when you go out and for how long while your lady is pregnant, it is indeed a good idea to get out of the house with your friends for some bonding time. Go blow off some steam via a basketball game with the guys, a round of beers at the pub, or what have you. Just don't go being irresponsible: don't drive drunk, and be sure to come home sober so you can continue to help out. But getting some breathing room helps you keep your act together around the house, so do it.

you with the tools to help her, and yourself, get through this tough time.

Help with her exhaustion by offering foot rubs and taking over chores when it comes to the house or anything else that you can lend a hand with. If you haven't done so already, get into the habit of splitting up responsibilities when it comes to the home. Allotting chores and responsibilities now will only make life easier when the due date arrives.

From this point on, you have to adjust to the new dynamic your little one will bring to your lives. You can never be over-prepared, but at the same time you will ultimately just need to experience it for yourself to figure out what works best for you and your partner. Know that it is going to be chaotic for a bit. That's normal. That's parenting.

TELLING THE REST OF THE WORLD

Now that you know baby is on the way for sure and you've told your family, how to break the news to your buddies and coworkers.

Now that you've figured out how to survive trimester one, you're probably itching to share the good news (if you haven't already). Around three to four months in, you are entering the safe zone and feeling more confident. By "safe zone" I mean that the chances of a miscarriage reduce after the first trimester, so you can more safely start to share the news if you choose to. You've held off on telling the general public for this long. You've leaked the news to your folks, but now it may be time to tell your friends, coworkers, and acquaintances. Who and when to tell should be a joint decision you make with your partner.

Once you decide to spread the word, how do you share it? Decide together how you will share the news. We didn't have the luxury of social media for any of our three pregnancies. Not even cell phones. We told people the old-fashioned way: the home telephone. Today you have the option to share the announcement through the news feed on your own personalized website. You can let everyone and anyone know in a matter of seconds! But use your due diligence when you decide who you're gonna tell—and how.

Telling friends can be a bit nerve-wracking, as part of you is psyched while the other part may be scared you will be excommunicated from your posse. But there's no hiding the fact that you are having a kid, so while you may be able to get away with not telling your buddies until the last minute, don't think they won't get suspicious when all of a sudden you are not around much anymore with no explanation at all. Plus, they may think you were a bit of an a-hole for not telling them. "*That's* what's been making you so edgy these last coupla months? Well, duh!" Dude, they are your friends. They will eventually accept and embrace your new role or they won't. If they don't . . . are they actually good friends? If your single (or childless) friends can't relate to you once you become a dad, then here's a news flash: they are not meant to be in your life much longer. Seriously. It doesn't mean you shouldn't talk to them, it's just that you will have less to talk about and relate to.

Of course, once you do start to share the news, you'll find that not everyone is skilled when it comes to communicating this sort of thing, so keep that in mind and temper your expectations when it comes time to share. Not everyone is going to automatically jump for joy, light a cigar, and pat you on the back for a job well done. For instance, when my wife told her grandmother she was pregnant, her grandma's response was "Oh dear. I can't picture you being a mom." Grandma meant no disrespect, but this was *not* the reaction Meredith was expecting. She got upset, but instead of trying to change her emotions about the situation, I was able to listen and to be disappointed too and to validate her feelings. In hindsight it seems easy, but I must admit it's not my first instinct with my wife. I typically want to take the discomfort away by offering solutions. Try this next time you find yourself in a similar situation. You will find it really works.

When you do decide to announce the good news, there are creative ways to spill the beans. I have some friends who decided to use their shower to announce the gender of their baby. It was a surprise for everyone, even them. They decided not to

> ## → THERE ARE NO SOCIAL MEDIA DO-OVERS
>
> One thing to keep in mind with social media (and it's something I repeatedly share with my kids in our household): once you put it out there you can't take it back. So, Dad, if you are thinking of Tweeting a photo of your wife's belly, the first sonogram, or even a comedic phrase like "Guess who's knocked up?" or "Looks like my boys can swim!" be sure you clear it with the wife. After all it's her body you're posting about. It would suck to start off the announcement of her pregnancy with an embarrassing cyber moment that you can't take back.

find out during the ultrasound and instead asked the doctor to write down the sex of their baby on a piece of paper. They then took the slip of paper to the bakery that was catering their event. Only the doctor and the baker knew what the sex of the baby was. Personally, I don't have the patience to wait that long, but to each his own.

I have to say, it was a damn tasty cake.

And it turned out to be a girl!

THE FRIENDSHIP GAME

How to deal with friends that aren't as accepting of your new role, and how to meet new ones.

It is important for you to maintain your friendships as best you can while embarking on this new path. There will be times

when you want a friendly ear, when you are feeling overwhelmed with the stress of pregnancy or the oncoming birth.
It's healthy to acknowledge that fear is a normal part of parenting. Dealing with the changes that occur in your relationship
during pregnancy is best handled when you are able to express
these feelings to a friend who is willing to listen and understand. Get into the habit early on of finding the support you
need, someone you can vent to, blow off some steam with, and
get some perspective from on what you are experiencing. Support for both of you—as a couple and as individuals—is necessary. Stick with those who share your joy.

When we became parents the first time around, when it
came to our childless friends, we felt like we experienced a
death to a certain degree. Part of us didn't relate to them
anymore; our schedules were totally off, and our priorities had
changed. Some friends got it and some didn't. A moment sticks
out in my mind when my wife and I couldn't attend a friend's
birthday dinner because her husband was sick with a stomach
virus. We regretfully declined and explained that between my
wife's compromised immune system and our newborn baby,
there was no way we were going to risk entering that environment. They absolutely could not understand our point of view.
Chances are you'll encounter similar situations, so addressing
early on with your friends your potential unavailability over
the coming months can help avoid hurt feelings down the line.

While some of your existing friendships may change, once
you officially announce your pregnancy status, you will soon
discover a new world of friendships. It's kinda cool. You'll meet
people in line at the grocery store, during parenting classes,
or while taking a stroll through the hood. These people can
end up becoming your new inner circle. In fact, many of our

closest friends today are folks we met through our babies, and we've remained close as we've watched our children grow up together. Of course, as kids get older they gravitate toward their own friendships, so you may transition in and out of friendships with their parents, but the friends of yours that really matter will stick around regardless of whether your kids are on the same soccer team or not that season. And believe me, in the coming months, you will definitely want friends to lean on as you deal with the emotional whirlwind that is her hormonal imbalance.

HORMONES, HORMONES, HORMONES

Her body is in a state of flux, so you need to be the steady one.

Can you imagine if we men had to take on the challenge of hormones like our female counterparts? Picture your worst night out drinking, where you can't function the next day so you get caffeinated to slog through. *That* is what it's like for many pregnant women for months and months. Imagine what life would be like in that state all the time. Plus, your wife has to go to work, deal with you, *and* manage all the physical stuff happening to her body.

I vividly recall walking into our kitchen one morning to discover my wife sobbing. Immediately I assumed the worst— someone had died or was in the hospital. When I asked my wife what happened, she simply pointed to the refrigerator, where we had posted the image of the first sonogram. Now, that picture had been up from the moment we got home from our doctor visit, yet here she was a few weeks later with tears streaming down her face. Why?

Hormones.

Moments like that occurred quite often with my wife. In fact, when I recently asked her to recall some specifics, she said that she remembers "crying over everything, from the joys and the sorrows of the world to the trash not being taken out." Now, if *that* doesn't explain how intense those chemical messengers are, then I don't know what does. Keep this in mind when you are attempting to navigate the explosions. Sometimes you will just have to surrender. This advice is not meant to emasculate you in any way. Instead, it's about knowing how to gracefully pick and choose your battles, and for the most part, choosing not to argue.

Extreme mood swings are another side effect you need to be prepared to handle, and it's not just hormones that cause them. Mood swings during pregnancy can be triggered by mental and physical stresses, fatigue, and changes in her metabolism, or by changing hormone levels. Mood swings are generally experienced during the first trimester, between six to ten weeks, and then again in the third trimester, as her body preps for birth. The best way to describe this experience is to tell you to imagine walking through a minefield. At any moment you can take the wrong step and BOOM! You want to navigate through this minefield as best you can, but when you step on a land mine and are about to go up in flames, accept it. Your fate is inevitable, so just wait until the fire dies down and keep on moving forward as best you can.

Somewhere around the end of the first trimester and going into the second, women's senses get heightened, another effect for which you can thank hormones. In many cases, it's progesterone that is instigating the edge she seems to have in abundance these days, while estrogen is causing all the spirit. Meanwhile, her smelling skills will be super enhanced, so your manly musk may force her to drive ice picks into your eyeballs if you don't ease back. Suddenly, smells she once loved, she hates. Food she loved repulses her. Keep that in mind next time you come home with smelly take-out or forget to put your dirty clothes from the gym in the laundry. And be sure to cut down (if not cut out entirely) your cologne/aftershave if you wear that stuff. Though her smelling powers can weaken after the first trimester, each case is individual, so it's best to be considerate from the start. Limit the odors you introduce into the environment, from cologne to cooking to laundry.

Every woman responds differently to hormones. Some women experience heightened emotions, both good and bad, while others feel anxiety or depression. She is wearing her

> ### ➤ WONDERFUL WORLD OF HORMONES
>
> Big changes in her hormone levels during pregnancy can affect her level of neurotransmitters (brain chemicals that regulate mood). For many women, moodiness flares up at around six to ten weeks in, eases up in the second trimester, and then reappears as their pregnancy winds to a close. But it's not just Mom. According to neuropsychiatrist Louann Brizendine, author of *The Male Brain*, although men may not be aware of it, they too undergo hormonal changes as they prepare for fatherhood. For instance, levels of a stress hormone called Cortisol—the ol' fight-or-take-flight chemical—often increase six weeks in.

emotions on her sleeve throughout her pregnancy for sure though, so pay attention to what triggers her frustrations and anxieties, and what can potentially set her off, whether it's family, certain friends, political events, the closing of her favorite restaurant, her boss, whatever. Being aware of those triggers will inform you how to prevent moments of discomfort for both you and your partner.

Remaining curious, open, and nonreactive will serve you from this point on. Once your baby arrives, the real chaos begins, so you want to be a strong team by that point—work hard at it. Establishing your emotional language before you add another person to the mix will minimize the frustration of misunderstandings later. Not to say they won't happen. They will, be sure of it. So being skilled at handling those moments is what parenting is all about. By the way, I didn't learn this on my own. My wife often challenged me to improve my skills in these departments. Don't be fooled by stereotypes. We are all capable of being great communicators. Even in the stickiest of situations . . .

THE PORCELAIN THRONE
(AKA YOUR WIFE'S NEW BEST FRIEND)

Morning sickness kicks into high gear, the subtle art of vomiting, and what you can do to help avoid the mess.

Oh, morning sickness, how you vex us all. First off, they really should call it "mourning" sickness because, at its worst, your wife can feel like she's dying, and you will mourn the loss of your once cheerful partner. Plus the name is misleading because it's hardly relegated to the morning. She may feel sick in the morning, afternoon, mid-afternoon, early evening, nighttime, late night, and early morning. She may vomit often,

---

➤ MORNING SICKNESS TIPS

Some ways for her to cope with morning sickness include:

- Lie down. If she seems nauseous or dizzy, get her to kick those heels up and take a rest.

- Leave work. Her boss should understand if she needs to take a breather from the workplace.

- Sniff a fresh scent. When she can't pop open a window, encourage her to take a whiff of some enjoyable fresh scents. Lemon extract and peppermint oil are a good thing for her to carry in her purse.

- Vitamin B6 at 50 milligrams per day has been proven helpful. Consult with your doctor.

- Stay hydrated. Water is key.

- Find foods or drinks that ease nausea. Snacks like crackers or dry-roasted nuts, while drinks like flat Coke, 7UP, or seltzer with a slice of lemon, lime, or orange are said to help.

- Graze. Try to get her to eat up to six small meals a day rather than three big ones. Think small but frequent amounts. Have her stash food everywhere she might go throughout the day, such as the bathroom, bedroom, car, office, and so on.

- Ginger is her friend. Be it cooked, spiced, candied, raw, or in ale form, ginger is a good thing.

- Adjust her computer. Tone down the brightness, as the strobing can drive her nuts. Try it with her phone too (plus, it saves battery life).

- Carry a survival kit that includes water, vitamins, acid reflux meds, and even bowel stimulants.

and if you are really cool, you will offer to hold her hair while she heaves. I know, I know . . . the things we do for love . . .

Though there are many reasons why women feel nausea during pregnancy, a typical one is a decrease in blood sugar levels while they sleep. Though for some women nausea and vomiting begin right away, they usually start around the sixth week of pregnancy and are among the first signs that she's knocked up. Nausea can occur at any time of the day, and for most women it seems to stop around twelve weeks in. Some lucky women don't experience nausea at all. ("Who are these people?" my wife wonders.)

Along with helping ease your partner's nausea, you should also you familiarize yourself with the signs of serious complications from morning sickness. In extreme cases women can experience a condition known as hyperemesis gravidarum, a delightful complication highlighted by nausea, vomiting, weight loss, and dehydration. Mild cases are treated with dietary changes, rest, and antacids. More severe cases do require a hospital stay so that Mom can receive fluid and nutrition through an IV. Definitely consult your doctor if you fall into this atypical category.

Sometimes we men can feel powerless over our partners'

symptoms. No matter how strong we think we are, there is nothing we can do to change what is happening to her. We can, however, do everything in our power to make her more comfortable during this time. Consider *this* your contribution for the next nine months. It doesn't always have to be grand gestures either. We can do little things to ease their pain as well. One friend I spoke to said that he placed peppermint candles around the house and lit them around the clock to help ease his wife's nausea. I made it a point to shop for odorless food because the smells of certain things were driving my wife nuts. I have a friend whose wife was really suffering throughout her pregnancy, even resorting to sleeping on the couch, the only place she could find comfort enough to nod off. My friend felt so guilty sleeping with the bed all to himself that he crashed on the living room floor many nights just to be by her side. Sleeping next to your sick wife can be a great way to support your teammate!

SNACKS FOR MOM

Sour fruits, ginger, and mint are sources of relief for some women. When the dry heaving starts, having a supply on hand will make you a hero. While you're at it, dry salted crackers and/or soda water are also helpful in curbing nausea. If you're lucky, you may be able to get her to eat a simple pasta dish with a light sauce, olive oil, and salt, or a light tomato sauce. Dehydration often sets in at this time, so encourage drinking plenty of water. Keeping bottles or pitchers on hand throughout your home is smart, serving both as a reminder and relief.

COPING WITH SUPERPOWERS 'N' MOOD SWINGS

How to deal with the fact that pregnant women develop ultrasensitive senses that could destroy entire cities . . . and you.

Navigating through the first trimester of her pregnancy will take skill and flexibility on your part. If Bruce Lee were available to impart his martial arts skills, he would tell you that you must think like a warrior and be ready at a moment's notice for a surprise attack. You'll need the strength to take it like a man and the tolerance to not fight back.

First and foremost you need to take a deep breath the moment you sense your partner is acting out of the ordinary. Bear in mind that there is as much stress going on internally for her (even if she is not yet in touch with it) as there is for you: responsibility for the health of the baby, your future, your relationship, and so on. The same issues you are experiencing will surely be on the forefront of her mind as well. Being aware of this alone can really put things into perspective—you're both going through a lot of the same stress, just reacting in different ways.

➤ DIZZY MISS LIZZY

Pregnancy causes Mom's blood vessels to dilate and her blood pressure to drop, which can make her light-headed or dizzy. So if she looks like she's spacing out, grab that lady a chair!

Second, do not take her behavior personally. She's had to adjust her whole life in preparation for this baby. You have nine months to get your act together for your kid, while her life has changed in a matter of moments. Her hormones will be around for quite some time, so it's your job to be her coach and ground her when anxiety takes over. Having a heightened sense of awareness will be your best bet when these mood swings surface. It won't be an easy task. If you're anything like me, your first reaction when attacked is to defend yourself. But that behavior will only get you into trouble now. Listening is another skill that will serve you well during these emotional times. Being available to simply hear what she is experiencing without any judgment can give her some relief. You'll also want to practice patience. Take into consideration that your partner is dealing with many physical changes that may be difficult for her to accept. She is also insecure as hell about her looks these days, so making sure to compliment her and keeping your intimate side available will help ease her concerns during this time.

Mood swings don't always mean anger or irritability. Your partner can experience high times too. Well, not the kind of high you may be thinking. But she may feel sudden bursts of elation or joy about the impending arrival. These are the times you will want to just go along for the ride. But be prepared that she may shift to a supreme low just as quickly. These are the moments where you need to snap into your ninja warrior role to be of assistance.

At the end of the day these tips aren't solely for use during pregnancy. If you can make them a daily part of your life, your relationship will become more fluid and easier to navigate. Being in tune with your partner facilitates a deeper and

---

> ### DINNER DATES
>
> Since this is a delicate time in pregnancy due to nausea and vomiting, keeping it simple is the key. Most likely, a home cooked meal is the last thing your partner will desire. Try smoothies and juices as a good source of nutrition. Plain rice and chicken broth are also excellent, as they are quick, easy, and bland. Remember, at this stage keeping it simple is key!

---

more meaningful relationship. And speaking of deep and meaningful . . .

SEX: WILL WE EVER HAVE IT AGAIN?

Will she want to have sex when she's pregnant . . . and what do I do if she does?

"So . . . um . . . dude . . . like, can we still . . . ?"

Yes, sir.

You can still do it.

As long as your pregnancy is proceeding healthfully, you can have sex as often as you like. You may have to limit your positions to what she is comfortable with more so than normal. It's possible she could have cramps, abdominal pain, or even light contractions during or after sex. Have no fear. They are not caused by you per se, but rather the situation. Consider them false alarms, not powerful enough to start labor unless it's very close to her due date. In fact, doctors sometimes advise

> ━━━▶ WHAT IF . . .
>
> Penetration and vibration will not harm your baby, as he or she
> is protected by her abdomen and the uterus's muscular walls.
> The amniotic sac and the strong muscles of the uterus protect
> the li'l one, and the thick mucus plug that seals the cervix helps
> guard against infection. In other words, your wang ain't gonna
> get near the kid. You're all clear.

not having sex during the third trimester, to prevent an early delivery. But on the flip side it can be a useful tool in getting the little dude out if he is loving his digs just a bit too much. Each case is unique, so you should definitely consult with your wife's obstetrician first. But continuing to have a sex life during pregnancy is healthy and will keep you connected, so DO IT!

Some guys get freaked out about the idea of sex during pregnancy. My friend was convinced that his penis might even touch the baby in the womb. I laughed, "Don't flatter yourself. You ain't *that* big!"

If you are really having a hard time with the idea of sex, talk to her. Keeping open communication with your wife helps to minimize the chance of either of you feeling inhibited. Voice your concerns ahead of time and work through them together so you can continue to feel connected to your partner both emotionally and sexually. Getting advice firsthand from your doctor is important here too. Don't be shy. Be proactive and don't let any questions go unasked. The more information you can obtain in this department the better.

My wife was *totally* into having sex during pregnancy—after the intense nausea subsided, that is. In fact, most women who are having a healthy pregnancy may continue to want to have sex right up until their water breaks or they go into labor. Why? Increased sex drive is usually due to increased blood flow. That extra blood flow to her pelvic area can even cause engorgement of the genitals, resulting in a heightened sensation that can actually add to her pleasure during sex. Nature wants you to enjoy yourselves.

With that said, let her take the lead. Staying tuned in to your partner's transformation and letting her feel empowered is important when it comes to sex during pregnancy. The fact that you are even thinking about this subject is a good thing. Sex is obviously an important part of your relationship. Think of it this way: right now your partner is the thermostat, and you need to take her temperature. Her body is changing, and just like she gets cravings for food, she gets cravings for sex.

▸ DID YOU KNOW?

About two-thirds of a teaspoonful of seminal fluid is released on average during ejaculation, containing about 210 to 525 million sperm. About one-quarter of these sperm will be abnormal, but the remaining three-quarters will be capable of the independent movement that is needed to reach the fallopian tube. Once the sperm enter the vagina, they can be prohibited from continuing on their path by slightly acidic vaginal secretions. Of the millions of sperm released in each ejaculation, only a few hundred will reach the female egg in the fallopian tube. But it only takes one to do the job.

I would like to propose a new word to consider when it comes to sex during pregnancy: intimacy. After they've been together for a while, couples tend to fall into patterns regarding sex. Always at night, always after they've brushed your teeth, always the same position, or whatever. Start breaking those patterns now, buddy. This is good advice for your sex life in general when you have been with the same person for several years, but it is especially vital during pregnancy, when you ain't getting it enough and she is feeling unsexy yet horny. Start being intimate again, mix things up, and bring some romance and spontaneity back into the bedroom. Keeping your sex life fun and interesting is good advice for any relationship, but it is especially important now. Her body is changing, she is often feeling unattractive, and her ego is about as deflated as it's ever going to get. Therefore she needs as much positivity, complimenting, and physical attention as you can give her. Nothing will make her feel attractive more than the man in her life giving her that all-too-familiar "I need you right now" gaze and leading her into the bedroom.

As guys, we have it so much easier when it comes to sex. Think about it. For us orgasms can be achieved quite easily. That's not always the case for your partner. Most likely the two of you have already found your rhythm in your sex life. But now she's pregnant and you're gonna have to learn a new dance. The most important piece of advice I can recommend to you in this department is do not take it personally if she's not in the mood.

Be open and communicate ways you can fulfill each other's sexual needs, whether it's masturbation, toys, or oral sex. Be creative to stay connected. Start simple with cuddling in bed or rubbing her achy spots. Keep expectations low, just be together, and see where it goes. Depending on where she is at in her pregnancy, she may just be thinking, "How the hell do I get rid of this nausea?" and need a distraction. If she's further along or lucky enough to not suffer the pangs of nausea, then you may be in luck. But you need to ask in order to receive. Just make sure to give her body time to heal *after* delivery (four to six weeks) before you leap right back into your wild sexy ways.

What if you are the one who's experiencing a loss of interest? Communicate to your partner that she's not responsible. Share your needs and concerns with her in an open and loving way. And if talking about it doesn't open up the floodgates, and sex is unappealing, then try other forms of contact, like making out, cuddling, kissing, or massages. You can also try leaving each other sexy texts, selfies, phone messages, or emails to get each other hot and bothered throughout the day, so that sex is a must when you get home. Nothing like a slow burn to make a raging fire!

Remember . . .

- By the end of the first trimester the baby has formed and is in her tummy.

- It's okay to start telling the world about your good news, if you are comfortable with that.

- Some friends will be supportive, others will not, new ones will arrive.

- Her mood swings are a-swingin'. Try to understand what she is going through.

- When she is getting irritable, take a deep breath, don't take it personally, and listen. Her senses get heightened, so she might get annoyed with things that didn't bother her before.

- There may be vomiting or morning sickness. It's perfectly normal. Be there for her.

- Have no fear: many women still want to have sex after becoming pregnant, some more than ever.

CHAPTER

2

The Second Trimester

So here we are at the start of the second trimester. Only 180 more days, give or take, until the little bundle of joy and terror arrives. Hopefully you and your partner still feel close as a couple and the mood swings and nausea haven't gotten the best of you. As you enter this second phase of her pregnancy, many of her symptoms, including nausea, can disappear for a while. But don't worry, there will be plenty of new symptoms to look forward to, like her need to pee more than ever and her cravings for very specific foods.

This is also the phase where her body will begin to change . . . noticeably. Her tummy is starting to swell, her breasts are getting bigger, and she's gaining weight. You need to start tending to her, bro. We will discuss things you can do to help ease the pain and get her to relax. More than anything else, you need to be supportive.

While your wife will still be going through a lot of changes during this time, make sure to celebrate what brought you together as a couple in the first place. Planning a getaway for a few days together is something you should take advantage of if your wife is feeling better and you can afford it. Even an overnighter can be enough to give your love life a little boost during this time. Try to not let the pregnancy completely dismantle your sex or social life. Getting back into your element (your groove, if you will) and focusing on each other now is important, especially since it will become more difficult once your little one is in the picture.

WRAPPING YOUR HEAD AROUND ALL THIS

Your baby is on the way, your mind has been blown, please proceed . . .

Before we get into the nitty-gritty of what is happening to your partner's body and how you fit into all of that, let's address the fact that this is all a lot for you to take in. You may be feeling anxious, nervous, or a little freaked out. The tone of the second trimester is noticeably different. The reality has set in. The clock is ticking. Her emotional changes are coming just as fast as the physical ones, and you're not always sure what is a real issue versus a randomly activated mood swing. This is normal. Just like when you first got to know her, you will suss out all her quirks and triggers and learn to deal with (or avoid) them. Be aware that she is ultrasensitive for a while, so tread lightly.

> ──▶ **DID YOU KNOW?**
>
> Your baby is about the size of a large plum and has his or her own unique fingerprints around thirteen weeks. At fourteen weeks your baby can smile and frown, while at fifteen weeks baby can make facial expressions and can even suck his or her thumb.

This is not the time to be lashing out emotionally when you are frustrated or feel pressured.

In fact, rather than letting this phase alienate you from your partner, use this opportunity get closer with her, to bond more. Instead of bottling up the feelings that need to be communicated, try opening up and expressing yourself. Communicate. Erupting out of anger or frustration just makes the situation worse.

If the time comes when you find yourself letting it all fly without a filter, reel yourself back in before it's too late. Talk *with* her, not *at* her. Let her know how you feel in a calm, open manner. Once you get that weight off your chest, you can be honest without the fear of hurting her (or maybe you already did) and really get to the bottom of any lingering issues. Then, you can kiss and make up. And we all know the best part of fighting is make-up sex anyways, so let nature take its course.

It still amazes me how complex we humans are, especially during pregnancy. The fact that my sperm was part of the transformation that my wife experienced was mind-blowing. How the hell a sperm and egg turn into an embryo that forms into a baby is beyond me. During the second trimester, take time to appreciate the miracle of this process (scientifically, religiously, or however you slice it—it's still a friggin' miracle). The last thing you want to do is take for granted how important this experience is, and will be. I only wish I had stayed more in the moment during all three of my wife's pregnancies. I recall feeling overwhelmed with the responsibilities and not knowing if I could handle this transition financially, emotionally, or physically. Focusing on those triggers can create an enormous amount of anxiety and it's almost impossible to avoid. To distract yourself and manage anxiety, focus on your partner and staying in the moment. Take baby steps. One foot at a time.

Since your partner's body is changing more dramatically during this time, the reality of the pregnancy is really going to settle in. Not all of us dudes are in touch with how to handle this. When my wife was expecting our first, I had no other guy friends in my boat. Hopefully the same is not true for you. A solid support system of bros that you can lean on is a comforting thing. Fight the stereotype that men are unwilling to seek help or emotional comfort from other men. Bottling up your

---

> **DID YOU KNOW?**
>
> Week twenty-four is one of the major milestones of pregnancy. At this point, your baby is classified as "viable"—that is, he or she would stand a good chance (around 39 percent) of surviving if born now. Baby also has his or her own daily waking and sleeping patterns by this time. Unfortunately, they may not tie in with your partner's, so watch out!

fears and anxieties inside will not serve you in the end. Find a network of guys to share your experience/fears and reduce your anxiety tremendously. Today I am fortunate to have a close group that I meet with once every few weeks for drinks, to catch up and shoot the shit. Almost every time we hang, we end up sharing our challenges, fears, and joys in parenting and marriage. I can't encourage you enough to reach out to people who can help you dialogue about what you are going through and provide you with feedback, during and beyond pregnancy. It really helps to have a sounding board when you hit those major milestones of parenting.

ULTRASOUND:
THE MUST-SEE MOVIE OF THE YEAR!

Those ghostlike X-ray images of your
child and what they mean.

If there is one film you must see this year, it is her sonogram. Think of it as being nominated for Best Ultrasound of the Year at the Oscars, so you better damn well show up and accept that award! And chances are you will know ahead of time when your first ultrasound appointment will take place, so there really are no excuses for not being there. This kind of stuff gets scheduled in advance with her doctor, so stay in tune with what is going on.

Most women have two ultrasounds during their pregnancy. The first occurs in the first trimester (between six and ten weeks) to confirm that she is pregnant. This is when you see the baby for the first time and they determine the due date.

KEEP THAT BLOOD SUGAR LOW, BABY

Around week twenty-four (the milestone week we just mentioned), the mother will need to undergo a glucose screening
test, which is essentially a blood exam that tests for gestational
diabetes, a high blood sugar condition related to pregnancy.
This test can freak a lot of women out because untreated or
poorly controlled gestational diabetes can hurt the baby. However, knowledge is power, and early diagnosis and careful
monitoring by your doctor can help keep your baby safe and
healthy.

Then in the second trimester (around eighteen to twenty
weeks), another ultrasound takes place to check the baby's
anatomy and to screen for developmental abnormalities. Be
sure to mention ahead of time if you do not want to know the
baby's sex.

The first ultrasound can be a bit of a nerve-wracking experience. The day of Meredith's first ultrasound was particularly
stressful since we were nervous about being newcomers to pregnancy *and* concerned over the health of the baby and my wife.
Thinking we were classified as high-risk scared us big-time,
and we went in holding our breath from the get-go. I don't
think I would have ever appreciated how emotionally complex
this visit could be if I had not been there to experience it myself. My wife needed my support, and your partner will need
yours too.

That being said, seeing the image of my baby for the first
time was one of the most exciting experiences of my life. That
black-and-white image of little Kai blew my mind. It was even

cooler when we saw the second ultrasound a few months later (doctors recommend a routine second trimester ultrasound just to make sure everything is moving along smoothly) and he had started to really look like a little person. We could see arms, legs, and even tiny fingers!

SEX STATUS

*Do you want to know? To be or not to be
(a boy or a girl), that is the question.*

A sonogram is a noninvasive diagnostic test that uses sound waves to form a visual image of the baby, placenta, uterus, and other pelvic organs. This prenatal ultrasound gives the doctor valuable information about the progress of the pregnancy and the baby's health. Your partner will have an ultrasound around six to ten weeks to confirm the pregnancy and get the due date. The standard mid-pregnancy ultrasound takes place between sixteen and twenty weeks in, and that is when you'll likely learn the baby's sex if you choose. Normally, doctors can determine the baby's sex during that mid-pregnancy ultrasound, but not always. Sometimes the boy's penis is tucked behind, so the doctor can't tell for sure, or the baby is just in a weird position that makes it tough for the doctor to see details. As a result, many parents don't find out the sex until several months later.

Determining the sex of your child ahead of time is a sensitive issue. It's totally subjective, and I am not here to tell you knowing is better than not. But what I can say is that it is a topic that you want to make sure you both agree on, so don't wait until that ultrasound appointment to figure out what you are going to do.

Meredith was convinced our first child would be a girl until we found out otherwise from the ultrasound. She asked the doctor if he was 100 percent sure and he responded, "I will pay for the college education of this child if I am wrong." Damn, that was the only time I was disappointed with the results.

For me, it felt useful to know ahead of time so I could avoid any disappointment at delivery time if I was hoping to have a boy and it turned out to be a girl (or vice versa). In fact, the moment we found out the sex of our first (and second and third) child, we began calling our baby by the name we had chosen. It seemed unnatural for us not to speak to our children as if they were already born, especially since babies can

➤ BABY GEAR

The second trimester is a great time to think about all the gear and necessities you will need once your baby arrives. Luckily there are tons of websites at your fingertips to advise and suggest what you will need the moment the birth occurs (see "Baby Showers and You" in Chapter 3 for some tips). We didn't have the luxury of such easy cyber-browsing when we had our kids, so my wife and I did it the old-fashioned way. From Babies "R" Us to Buy Buy Baby, you will be able to find everything you will possibly need and tons of crap you won't. Getting involved in shopping for baby is a fun way to connect and can help to bridge any gaps of disconnect you may feel by this time.

hear while in the womb, as early as eighteen weeks. Interestingly, doing this helped me to feel a closer connection to each of our children, since I was speaking to them by name and sharing stories of things I wanted to do with them once they were born. It made me more excited at the prospect of becoming a dad.

Finding out the sex ahead of time can also eliminate the stress of planning the nursery, painting rooms, buying clothes, and so on. Of course, to be safe you can choose to do these things in a gender-neutral color. I guess it really depends on what personality type you are. If you think about it, before we were so technologically advanced, there was no accurate way to tell what the gender of your child would be. People relied on old wives' tales like pulling down the skin under your left eye to look at the white part of your eyeball. They say if you see a vein that looks like a V or branches, you are having a girl. Okay, that one is just plain crazy. Can you imagine how many scores of women who were relying on that tale were surprised once they delivered? The point is, people did just fine before they had all of this modern technology and information.

Bottom line, if you are a man hell-bent on having a son, then I suggest you find out the sex of your baby ahead of time. The last thing your partner will want to see is a disappointed face after going through the pains of labor. Of course, I can't imagine anyone being disappointed after going through all that, but you never know. If the baby's sex is that important to you, you can always keep trying until you get what you were hoping for. I know a couple who desperately wanted a boy, yet three girls later there was still no li'l dude in sight. At some point, they just gave up on the notion of having a son. Those three girls are terrific though, and the parents can't imagine their life any differently now. Some things are just meant to be. No matter what, you will love your kids and want to connect with them.

SOME FOOD ADVICE FOR MOM

You hear a lot of dos and don'ts about what she can and can't eat. Let's address a few.

At this stage in the game, once she felt up to eating again, my wife loved when I took the reins and made dinner plans out for us. Thankfully, once the second trimester began, she could finally get through a regular meal. Lamb chops were one of her major cravings, so I made it a point to throw some chops on the grill at least once a week. I was so relieved we could finally introduce our favorite foods and smells back into our life again. So take the initiative and plan out some tasty dinners ahead of time and surprise your lady.

However, there are some dos and don'ts regarding what she can and cannot eat while preggers.

With some exceptions (below), she can basically consume what she would normally eat. In fact, it is a myth that she should eat for two, by the way. A pregnant woman's calorie intake grows during pregnancy, but that doesn't mean she should double up on her meals. A mother's diet needs to be balanced and nutritious for a healthy pregnancy. This means finding the right balance of proteins, carbohydrates, and fats, and eating lots of vegetables and fruits. There are a few things she should avoid eating altogether though for a while.

She should definitely stay away from any type of unpasteurized milk and certain types of soft cheese during pregnancy as they run the risk of carrying a bacteria called Listeria. So no more Brie, Camembert, Roquefort, Feta, Gorgonzola, or Mexican-style cheeses, like queso blanco and quesco fresco. Some imported cheeses are made with pasteurized milk and are safe to eat, but be cautious with dairy in general. And speaking of bacteria, it is also best for her to stay away from deli meats such as bologna, salami, ham, turkey, and hot dogs unless they have been thoroughly heated and are steaming hot, as they can cause listeriosis, a type of food poisoning caused by the aforementioned Listeria.

So what's the deal with pregnancy and shellfish? Can she or can't she eat it and why or why not? First off, raw fish, like oysters and sushi, are a definite no-no as they can contain harmful bacteria or viruses. Sushi can also contain parasites such as tapeworms that, if they grow large enough, can rob her body of nutrients needed for the growing baby. However, unless your partner is highly allergic to it (and if she doesn't know, now is not the time to find out), eating cooked shellfish is okay. But Mom definitely needs to be conscious of the levels of mercury found in certain types of fish she consumes, especially tuna. Mercury during pregnancy has been linked to developmental delays and brain damage.

In general, discuss any nutrition and food concerns you have with your doctor ahead of time. The more you can learn about her health and nutrition needs the better.

CRAVINGS AND SYMPATHY (WEIGHT) FOR THE DEVIL

Work in workouts, but how much exercise can she handle?
And you need to get your act together, mister. Yes, YOU!

Pickles and ice cream. You've heard about it. You've seen it in cartoons and sitcoms. You pray it's a myth. Well, it is. Sort of . . .

About half the women in America report at least one food craving during pregnancy, says Judith Brown, author of *What to Eat Before, During, and After Pregnancy*. So it goes without saying that there's a chance your partner will get food cravings. For the most part though, they are not as unusual as TV leads you to believe. Sure, she may suddenly crave pickles and ice cream, but more likely she'll just want some fast food, fruit, or other fairly normal things. Your partner can definitely end up craving foods that she would otherwise not be caught eating in a million years. And chances are any strange cravings will end as soon as the pregnancy is over.

Meredith did have some interesting cravings during her pregnancy. With Juliette (our second), avocado with lemon and salt, and banana cream pie were top of her list. However, with Kai, she craved lamb chops and steaks constantly. This could've been due to an iron deficiency, I suppose, but either way, I was psyched. I am a total meat eater, so when these cravings came on it was my time to shine, baby!

Like most dudes I feared that once she got pregnant I would be forced to make those late night runs to the store for the aforementioned pickles and ice cream or whatnot, but thankfully, those desires never really kicked into overdrive. Meredith liked some stuff more than usual, and I was happy to get it for

> ───▶ **IMPORTANT SUPPLEMENTS**
>
> A list of key supplements she can take to stay healthy and energetic during pregnancy:
>
> - Water
> - Iron
> - Calcium
> - Vitamin C
> - Vitamin B
> - Vitamin D
> - Magnesium
> - Folic acid
>
> Plus, omega-3 and omega-6 fatty acids are recommended for the proper growth and development of the fetus.

her, but it wasn't like she was waking me at four in the morning demanding I go to 7-Eleven or anything. Of course, today we have the luxury of grocery delivery services, so if that late night craving set in and we were out of stock, a simple phone call would solve the problem.

There is no one reason to explain why women crave certain foods during pregnancy. Hormones are partly responsible, but not 100 percent. At the end of the day though, unless she's craving paint chips, laundry detergent, or dirt (otherwise known as a condition called pica, for which you should seek the advice of your doctor), there is no reason for her not to indulge in the cravings.

The trick is to balance letting her indulge along with making sure she eats right. What is eating right for a pregnant

> ### → FOOD TIPS AND CALORIES
>
> A mother's diet and lifestyle are key to producing the healthi-
> est baby possible. But she is not, as the myth says, eating for
> two, so don't let her overdo it. The reality is that she is eating
> for herself plus a very tiny person, so she really only needs to
> add an extra three hundred calories a day. Try working nutri-
> tious veggies and fruits into her diet, plus lots of lean protein
> and complex carbs. Have her try eating smaller meals (yes, you
> read that right . . . smaller) more frequently throughout the day
> too. Make sure she drinks lots of water, gets plenty of exercise,
> and don't let her deny herself a treat every so often . . . she's
> earned it!

lady? Well, protein contains amino acids that are an important
building block of human cells. Given the rapid cell development of your wee baby-to-be, protein should be an essential
part of Mom's pregnancy diet. She should aim for three serv-
ings of protein daily (adding up to about seventy-five grams),
and try to spread it out throughout the day. For example, a
cheese omelet for breakfast, a (cooked) salmon salad for lunch,
and a chicken breast with dinner is a fine way to go. She can
get additional protein from whole-grain breads and cereals,
and calcium-rich foods like milk and yogurt. What if she's a
vegan mama? Well, if she doesn't eat animal proteins, she can
ramp up her intake of vegetable source proteins such as grains,
legumes, and small amounts of fermented soy.

But here's the rub. While she is partaking in lamb chops
and cream pie, her trusty sidekick (that is, *you*) is also indulg-
ing in said deliciousness. Except you ain't even close to eatin'

for two, so your belly starts to grow too. And not in a good way! You'll be surprised by how quickly the pounds add up on you as well. So don't get carried away. Eating in moderation is always your best bet. But if you find that you seem to be getting out of hand with how much you are eating (or what you are eating), take it upon yourself to be a good partner and suggest foods that are similar in taste that may have fewer calories. Try, say, sorbet instead of ice cream to see if it satisfies her urge. Tasty yet less fattening.

But if you find that curbing cravings is just way too difficult, then perhaps finding a way to include exercising together can ease your guilt while working off the excess weight. My wife and I made it a point to take morning walks together once she had the energy to do so. I have some friends whose wives were

---

➤ BABY FOOD (NO, NOT *THAT* KIND!)

While there is no direct link between her cravings and the gender of your child, traditional wisdom states that craving protein-rich products can mean you are having a boy, while craving products that are sweet, like chocolate or fruits, can mean it's a girl. Interestingly, during my wife's lamb chop phase we ended up with a boy, and the banana cream pie craving resulted in a girl. Loose science to be sure. Meanwhile, both kids are lovers of the main craving their mom experienced during their pregnancy. So a popular Pegula family meal might consist of lamb chops, chips and guacamole, and banana cream pie for dessert. Go figure, right? Perhaps those old wives' tales stand for something after all.

avid runners and ran right up to the day they delivered. I kid you not! As always, make sure to check with your doctor, since every woman's pregnancy is individual. But unless your pregnancy is deemed high risk, some exercise will be advised, so put on your velvet seventies sweat suit and lace up your sneakers!

GO WITH THE FLOW

Catch up on her condition, what she needs from you, and what booby traps to avoid (literally!).

Again, the second trimester is when your partner's body will begin to change more dramatically, and if it hasn't already become real to you, it probably will now. During this period your baby continues to grow and develop. Hopefully you will too.

How exactly is your partner's body changing?

DID YOU KNOW?

Not only are the organs of the baby growing during the pregnancy, but some of Mom's organs grow too. Don't worry, it doesn't hurt her and it all goes back to normal after delivery. A steroid hormone called progesterone released during pregnancy softens the joints, so her rib cage stretches out as her uterus grows. Organs like the heart and liver enlarge too due to their extra workload, while everything else in her body shifts around as well.

Well, she's peeing. A LOT. Don't be a dick and ask her to hold it. Long trip or not, if she needs to go, you're pulling over! Why so much? Well, hormonal changes cause blood to flow faster through her kidneys, which fills her bladder more often. During the nine months of her pregnancy the blood levels in her body will rise until she has nearly 50 percent more than before. This means that lots of extra fluids are being processed through her kidneys and end up in her bladder. Hence, pee.

She also may experience some changes in the pigment of the skin on her face (called melasma, aka the mask of pregnancy) and/or down her abdomen. Stretch marks might become more noticeable too. Don't worry; these are standard symptoms of the second trimester.

During this time, she could experience feelings of being light-headed, which is caused by the dilation of her blood vessels due to hormone changes. Leg cramps can enter the picture, as well as the beginning of Braxton Hicks contrac-

---

➤ TIPS ON BRAXTON HICKS

Braxton Hicks contractions are intermittent uterine contractions often interpreted incorrectly as false labor. However, unlike real labor, there is no real pattern. They sometimes start around six weeks into a pregnancy and are also known as practice contractions. They can be triggered by dehydration, a full bladder, or being overly active, and usually last between fifteen seconds and two minutes. While they can start to occur as early as six week of pregnancy, they are most common after the second trimester.

tions (see box on page 59). Consider these warm-ups for the big-time contractions she'll face on delivery day, so empathize with her and see what you need to do to make her feel more comfortable.

One day during the second trimester, my wife asked me point-blank if she looked fat. Without hesitation I blurted out, "Gee, honey, it's hard for me to tell since I see you all the time." It was one of my rare moments of brilliance. There was no way in hell I was going to answer yes! Of course, she had indeed gained quite a bit of weight, but this was not the time to be *completely* honest about such things. We all know that in life there are times you simply have to lie to do the right thing. This is one of those times, dude! A few other good responses are "You always look beautiful to me," "Who can tell with that radiant glow," or "Fat? You look sexy!"

If your partner is feeling self-conscious about her changing body, consider giving her a light massage. (However, when you get to the third trimester, be sure to check with her doctor to make certain there's no chance of her going into labor from

---

➤ DID YOU KNOW?

Around the twentieth week, the uterus (the muscular organ that holds the fetus) can have expanded up to twenty times its normal size! By week twenty-two, baby is covered with a fine, down-like hair called lanugo that helps hold Vernix caseosa (that cheese-like white substance that coats newborn human babies) onto the skin. Your baby's eyebrows might be visible by this phase as well.

the rubdown!) Be it on her back, her neck, or her feet, a well-timed massage offer will score you major points. Rubbing cocoa butter on her belly or her thighs and legs can bring relief to both of you, and who knows, perhaps it can lead to something more.

... AND THEN THERE'S BOOBS

Many of you are thinkin', "Hey, I can deal with all these changes if I get to play with these big ol' porn star breasts!" Sadly this will not be the case.

What is it with our fascination with women's breasts? I mean, we know women generally enjoy a man's penis, yet we don't hear them commenting on 'em all the time, do we? Yet we men blather on incessantly about boobs to anyone who will listen and are generally obsessed with them (unless you're a butt man, of course . . . much respect). Bottom line is that for men, the fact that most women's boobs get bigger during pregnancy is an amazing and unexpected bonus.

Yet what is exciting to you is not so thrilling for her. Though they will grow substantially during pregnancy and, depending on if she breast-feeds or not, may remain that way for some time after, they don't feel all that terrific to the woman they adorn. Her breasts increase in size due to hormonal changes and increased blood flow. These changes can make her breasts feel sore, tingly, and unusually sensitive to the touch. Many women liken this to feelings they encounter before having their period. These changes can begin as early as four to six weeks into her pregnancy, but it's usually around six to eight weeks

---

TO SQUEEZE OR NOT TO SQUEEZE

Talk to her doc about the consequences of nipple stimulation.
I know, it sounds weird to say, but nipple stimulation has been
known to cause labor, usually only during the final stages of
pregnancy. So it's best to know what is and isn't good during
this time.

---

that the breasts begin to grow. Some women's breasts can grow
as large as a whole cup size. Whoa!

You'll also notice her nipples getting darker and the area
around the nipples (her areolas) becoming bigger as well. It's
all great fun for us men, but be mindful that the ladies can be
sore from all this upsizing. Oh, if only our penises grew larger
during pregnancy too, right? Wishful thinking . . .

It's in your best interest at this time to be supportive of your
partner by not cracking jokes or commenting to your friends
in front of her how she now has a rad new set of jugs. While I
don't discourage complimenting her on her recently acquired
attributes, don't go overboard. The last thing you want is to
set her up for discomfort and insecurity once she goes back
to her original pre-pregnancy, post-breast-feeding size. Also,
some women who have small breasts to begin with may feel
bummed out if their partner suddenly gets a little too psyched
now that they have such big ones. Be careful not to insult her.
Take her lead and let her be the one to make the comments.
All you need to do is stand by your gal and be proud. Let her
boobs speak for themselves. Hmmm . . . that didn't come out
right . . .

Once your partner has the baby, her breasts are likely to shrink back again. If she's lucky—and working out helps—her breasts will go back to normal, or possibly even retain some of their increased growth. By the time they're done breast-feeding though, many women's breasts have gone through the wringer and can sag. Meredith and I felt strongly about the baby getting nutrients straight from Mom to promote health and prevent disease, so we chose to let the forces that be take over and go the breast-feeding route, sag or not. Sadly, men's penises, and especially our scrotums, can do the same as we get older. It's just life, dude.

➤ BOOBS: MYTHS VS. FACTS

Myth: She can't breast-feed if she has big breasts.

Fact: Not true. Women with large boobs can indeed breast-feed successfully, though sometimes baby prefers others positions rather than being at the breast. Try the time-honored football hold, girls!

Myth: If she has small breasts, she won't make enough milk to breast-feed.

Fact: Bullshit. When it comes to breast-feeding, size doesn't matter. The amount of milk depends on the baby, not the size of the breast.

Myth: She can't breast-feed if she has flat or inverted nipples.

Fact: Not necessarily true. She can do exercises or wear breast shields to help control inverted nipples.

GETTING CONNECTED WITH THE BABY

Reading, singing, and talking to her stomach: cute or crazy?

When her body is changing because of the baby inside, she's going to become extremely connected to the child. She's the one carrying the little tyke and experiencing baby's kicks and movements. But just because you're not carrying the baby doesn't mean you can't connect with your kid-to-be. So far you've been more of a spectator than a participant, but now it's time to start stepping up your game and making that connection with the baby.

At twenty-three weeks your baby can actually hear your voice. The more you speak to your baby, the more familiar the child becomes with your voice, and the bonding begins. Some guys read stories, sing, play an instrument, or simply talk aloud. It may seem a little kooky, but it really is a cool way to get the baby familiar with your voice and presence, consciously or subconsciously. Plus, Mom thinks you are just dreamy to bother with such routines. Your partner won't necessarily ask you to do it, but believe me, there is nothing sexier than her man humming a tune or reading Elmo books to his unborn child.

At first, it felt slightly awkward to talk to Meredith's stomach, but I gave it a shot. I began a ritual of reading a children's book to Mer's belly. At first, there was no response. But night after night I kept the ritual up. Eventually I made up a song and started to sing it to her stomach. Finally, after about a week, I got a reaction from our little dude. It was unbelievable. While I sang my song, all of a sudden my son moved closer to my side of her stomach. It was remarkable, a moment I will never forget. From that point on every time he heard my voice,

> ➤ **THE AMNIOCENTESIS TEST**
>
> One of many delightful examinations she might go through during the second trimester is an amniocentesis, a prenatal test that collects info about your baby's health from a sample of amniotic fluid, the fluid that surrounds the baby In the uterus. Not all women take this test though. It is usually reserved for women over a certain age or if there is a known risk of Down syndrome or other such complications.

he responded with either a kick or a physical move to get closer to my voice.

As the weeks went on, I got obsessed with getting more responses from my son, so I began playing the piano to see his reaction. It was so much fun. In fact, once Meredith was really showing, Kai would roll over to my side of her belly whenever he'd hear my voice. Watching her stomach move was amazing, freaky, and unbelievable!

Some women aren't into that, and that's cool too. Either way, make sure you balance the time you spend at night with your kid-to-be and the time you spend on your wife-at-hand.

I've said it before, but another great way to bond with your baby and your wife is through massage. Meredith had a ritual of rubbing cocoa butter on her stomach at night, as many believe it helps eliminate stretch marks. I was happy to rub it on for her. It was a nice way to unwind at night and relax before nodding off. Plus, it gave me another excuse to feel the baby move around, and having her man rub her down made my wife feel sexy and loved.

These are just a few ideas to get you started on the road to bonding, but don't stop here. Be creative and don't judge yourself. You're beginning a whole new chapter in your life, so be curious and take risks.

STAYING CONNECTED WITH YOUR PARTNER

Be a teammate with your partner during her physical and emotional transformation.

Among the most challenging moments in our relationship have been those that occurred when pregnancy disrupted our daily routine. As I mentioned, in my early days of fatherhood I supplemented the income from my job as an out-of-work actor by starting a dog walking business.

While my days were pretty much business as usual, for Meredith that was hardly the case. She was in graduate school getting her master's in psychology, teaching at a local private school, and auditioning for commercials and both TV and film. But once the nausea beast reared its ugly head, she was virtually nonproductive.

It was a dramatic lifestyle shift for her to go from being so active to being virtually inactive. She experienced extreme cabin fever and longed for even the trivial kind of interactions we had with people throughout the day—a chat with the bank teller or sharing some tabloid gossip with the grocery checkout gal. She got resentful that I was able to continue functioning normally, not saddled by the weight and discomfort. "You get to have a life," she'd say to me. I, on the other hand, didn't quite see it the same way. I felt the strain of creating a successful career and providing for our future. The last thing on my mind was social interaction. In fact, there were many days I secretly wished I could trade places and stay home for the day . . . without the extraordinary levels of nausea, of course.

The lengths our better halves go to to have our children is quite a sacrifice. I often forget how easy I had it during Meredith's pregnancies. Sure, I was stressed about the financial responsibilities of being a parent, but she had the pressure of keeping our baby safe the entire nine months. You have to be aware of what your partner is experiencing because she's going through significant physical changes while you get the luxury of going on with your life. For instance, you get to drink alcohol and eat what you want throughout this if you choose. Think about if you had to give up all that fun stuff. While you can't actually go through the same journey that she is on, you can be there alongside her as a friend and lover. But it takes a little effort. Read up on what is happening to her and think of things you can do to make her life a little easier. Her energy levels will be lower than usual as she gets bigger, so rather than pushing her to keep up with you, maybe lower yours so you two are running at the same pace. It'll keep you on the same track.

With that in mind, try to implement some of the following suggestions into your daily, weekly, or monthly rituals. They'll help you stay connected to your partner during her pregnancy and will lay solid groundwork for the rest of your relationship.

Keep the Lines of Communication Open

I can hardly keep track of the number of times when I have misinterpreted a reaction from my wife and immediately withdrawn to protect myself. This cut-and-run approach to emotions and ego may have flown before, but with her heightened emotions, it ain't gonna fly now. And it won't work when you are trying to discipline a child. It's time to start owning up to your feelings and communicating them thoughtfully. Often, a simple statement to her acknowledging that you understand what she is upset about will make a huge difference. It takes mucho awareness and effort on your part, but if you can be honest and straightforward with your emotions, and calm down when you sense you are losing it or being short-tempered, you will both benefit.

Do Not Overreact

Taking a deep breath and evaluating what just happened before firing back will save your ass every time, dude. By nature, men are built to protect themselves. But we can fight that instinct, and there can be many benefits to doing so. If you find yourself in front of the firing squad, take a breath and chill. I'm not asking you to be a punching bag, but simply to *remember all that your partner is going through and give her a break.* Is it more valuable to be "right" or to be present and have a happy partner? More often than not, I chose being right, and let me tell you, it didn't serve me in the long (or short) run. Relationships are complex. Add pregnancy to the recipe and forget about it. Try to bring the focus back to simplicity. Listen, breathe, and take it all in, dude. *Sometimes lending an ear is all you need to do.* If there is ever a time in your life when silence can truly be golden, this is it.

Empathize with Your Partner but Don't BS Her

WARNING: DO NOT TELL HER YOU UNDERSTAND WHAT SHE IS GOING THROUGH. That's just a flat-out lie. We don't know what it's like and we never will, and to even say we do can be interpreted as condescending. Better to tell her that you can only imagine how much it sucks to go through what she is experiencing and that you're there to support her however you can.

Be Flexible

You are going to have to get used to changing plans at the last minute. Many a date night out was canceled due to Meredith feeling too ill. I'd feel bummed but would remind myself this wasn't the end of the world. These sorts of cancellations will occur more frequently than ever. It can happen with weekend getaway plans too. Those bastard hormones always get in the way! They made Meredith feel like shit, so it's no wonder she preferred to sleep off the discomfort. Don't take it personally. Unless you need to show up for dinner with the boss and your job is riding on attending, chillax. You'll be on a schedule soon enough once the little one is in the picture.

Be Instrumental Not Supplemental

Make no mistake about it, dude, you play an important role in this experience, especially when it comes to your pregnant partner. Take the initiative and let her know you are there to help her and even take over when need be. For instance, read up on your own to learn about what she is experiencing in her current pregnancy state. Educate yourself about her experience, ask questions, and decide on issues together. Going into pregnancy, I relied a lot on her knowledge. Only afterward did I realize that had I been more proactive, I wouldn't have struggled so hard to feel connected in this journey. Knowledge really is power, dude, and today there is a wealth of it available on the Internet, so start a-learnin'! Read this book, and then read five more!

Together Time

When you're relaxing around the house, try to do as many things together as possible. If your wife is into reading books about what's going on with her body, then join in. Or if you don't feel like doing homework, then find something you dig to read alongside her. Try giving each other little book reports before bed. Ask her some questions about what she learned. Let her summarize and share that experience so that you're being educated and bonding with her. Play cards or board games. Battleship or Connect Four are shockingly fun for two adults . . . even without booze! Or just simply watch TV together. Nothing like snuggling under a blanket together with a movie and a big bowl of popcorn.

These are just tips to serve as a launching pad for you. Try some out and see what else comes to mind. I can pretty much guarantee that if you don't put in the effort, you're not gonna enjoy the experience. You think your home life is hard now? Just wait until baby shows up. There will be no time for anything. That's why focusing on the two of you now needs to be a priority. Eventually it gets easier, but having a strong foundation will help balance the moments when things get overwhelming and out of hand. And those moments will happen. Often.

Remember . . .

- Be there for the ultrasound, as it's your first glance at your developing child.

- Her belly is showing and she has to pee a lot. Be forgiving. Her body is changing in other ways too, including enlarged breasts and weight gain.

- She is developing food cravings . . . and so might you be!

- Deli meats, shellfish, and some cheeses are a no-no.

- Despite the boobs getting bigger, they may not be for touching for a while.

- Connect with baby by talking, reading, or singing to Mom's tummy. The baby hears you, and Mom thinks you are rad.

- Stay connected with your partner by reading up on and talking to her about what she is going through.

CHAPTER

3

The Third Trimester

The third trimester is the final stretch, and the tenor changes from the previous few months. Although some of her old symptoms, such as nausea and exhaustion, may suddenly reappear, they won't last much longer. You will probably notice your partner beginning to slow down due to the size of the baby (and her belly!) at this point, so you're gonna really have to rise to the occasion. Start taking care of more things around the house, add chores to your list, start cooking more (or at least picking up more takeout), and be available and accessible.

It probably feels like you've been on a roller-coaster ride these past five or six months, but keep hanging on, as you are almost at the finish line. The third trimester of pregnancy can be physically and emotionally challenging for Mom as baby's size and position can make it hard for her to get comfortable.

Among the possible delights your lady will face during this time are continued breast growth, weight gain, contractions, backaches, shortness of breath, even more frequent urination, heartburn, swelling, vaginal discharge, spider veins, varicose veins, and hemorrhoids. Meanwhile, you are getting plenty of sleep and look and feel terrific. Not exactly fair, is it? So be aware that you have things pretty good while she feels like crap, and treat her accordingly.

Yet despite all of your new awareness and duties, it is important to maintain who you are throughout all this too. Continue to have a life, see your friends, and do what you like to do. Just be adaptable. If you love to BBQ and the smells are driving her crazy, move the grill across the lawn so the fumes don't waft inside. Or just go get pickup at a local rib joint for a while (and score extra points by bringing some back for her). If you love to crank your music loud, do it in your car. If you love to shoot pool with the guys, do it somewhere close when Mom is napping. If you are walking out the door to go play a pickup game, and she says she feels like shit, just call the guys and say you'll catch the next one. *But then make sure you damn well catch the next game.* Don't forget: it is still important that you get to have your fun. You can still be yourself and have a life, dude. You just have to adjust . . . and watch out for land mines.

WHAT TO DO WHEN SHE FEELS LIKE CRAP

How you can be the best while she feels at her worst.

The sheer quantity of times you will hear the phrase "I feel terrible" during the third trimester cannot be underestimated.

It was one my wife was far too used to, not only because of her pregnancy, but because of the lupus double whammy. There were many days when she could barely make it out of bed due to extreme fatigue coupled with the arthritic pain in her joints. Witnessing this day in and day out was extremely difficult for me. I felt even worse not being able to do anything to take the pain away. Eventually I learned that a simple massage to her back, legs, or shoulders was enough to distract her from the pain and help put her in a better mood. In uncomfortable, achy pregnancy moments, using this technique of distraction can help your partner feel much better and taken care of.

If she can tolerate the smell of cooking, now may be a good time to show her some of your talent in the kitchen (more on this below). If you really want to impress her, set the mood with romantic flowers and candles. Go the extra mile each day by pitching in with chores around the house. Granted the house's tidiness may be the last thing on her mind at this stage in the game, but at least you will earn points for offering.

Not everyone feels so bad during the third trimester though. In fact, this stage can be one of the most exciting for many women since birth is becoming a reality. The third trimester is usually the time when your gift registry is completed (something you may want to have a say in since you will be heading out with your little one in tow and will want to make sure your style is not sacrificed), your birthing classes are beginning (or finishing depending on how early you start), and the nesting phase is commencing.

During the third trimester, Mom can get unexpected bursts of energy. This is a good thing, but make sure she doesn't overwork herself. It's easy for her to get excited about gaining some renewed energy and forget that her stamina ain't what it used to be. My wife was obsessed with preparing the home for our son's arrival: finalizing our son's room, buying all the necessary supplies for his arrival, packing our overnight bag for the hospital stay, and reviewing our birthing class handbook to prepare for the big day.

One duty I was responsible for was figuring out my work schedule so I could be available for the first few weeks after our son was born. This was crucial. Today, many are fortunate enough to work for a company that supports paternity leave. But not everyone is so lucky. Make sure you can plan time off to spend with Mom and baby in those first weeks after delivery so you can help her with chores and meals.

MAKIN' DINNER FOR MOM

You are going to have to take over the cooking for a while, so here's some recipes and tips . . .

At this point, you should pretty much be in charge of preparing meals and doing the grocery shopping. Mom is going to

---

DID YOU KNOW?

During the first six weeks of this period your baby will more than double in size, growing from approximately 1.5 to 3.5 pounds. The heavier they get as time goes on, the more sore her back will become from carrying them. Just sayin' . . .

need to rest and stay off her feet, so get some easy to prepare recipes assembled or plan your pickup route food-wise. However, heartburn is typical during this time, so eating smaller meals, limiting spicy foods, drinking lots of water, and staying away from caffeine can all help her. Oh, and raw veggies can increase gas . . . soooo . . . uummmm . . . well, I think you can figure that one out. Cook her damn veggies or suffer the consequences!

Some dudes love to cook, so taking over ain't a big deal, but for many others the only male chef they want to see near their kitchen is that Swedish Muppet with the funny hat and exploding pies on TV. If you are of this ilk, then hop on the Internet and find some easy recipes to help keep her on track with a healthy balanced diet. You can type in just about any keyword with the word "easy recipe" next to it in Google and get some choices. Eating small meals frequently, rather than three big ones all the time, is also helpful if she struggles with heartburn and/or acid reflux.

Here are some easy ideas:

Preparing a bowl of oatmeal first thing in the morning is a subtle way to get her a dose of folic acid and iron, both of which are important to her diet. Top that sucker off with some blueberries, almonds (protein), and decaf coffee or herbal tea and you got yourself a tasty li'l breakfast.

If you happen to be around at lunchtime to prepare a meal, think about making a simple egg salad or hummus in a pita sandwich. It's a good source of protein (about 22g). While you're at it, make one for yourself too.

Dinner can be simple too. Prepare the meat of your choice on a kabob with some veggies, fruit, or whatever she desires.

→ **LEMON PARMESAN CHICKEN RECIPE**

My buddy's wife used to love this one so much she taught it to him for when she didn't want to deal. Now he has mastered it and many others.

- 1 pound chicken cutlets (works with boned chicken too)
- 1 cup parmesan cheese (it's a hard cheese, it's okay)
- ½ cup olive oil
- 1 cup lemon juice
- Garlic (to taste)
- Salt and pepper (to taste)

Preheat oven to 375, put the chicken and everything else in a glass dish (or whatever), cook for 15 minutes, turn over, and cook for another 10. Take out and let cool for a minute. Throw some greens with some olive oil and vinegar on the side. Bang—you're in.

This is a simple way to get her something full of protein and balanced with some veggies too. Plus, you get to grill and play with fire, which is always awesome, right?

GET YER ASS IN CLASS!

Why classes are good for the both of you . . . despite the fact that my wife and I didn't do them at all. Hypocrisy, hear me roar!

First off, let me just say that Meredith and I did not take classes when she was pregnant. We both felt confident that we knew how to breathe and relax because we were yoga addicts back in the day. In retrospect this was quite naive. Eventually it dawned on us that maybe we didn't know everything and could use some tips, so we took a crash course in Lamaze with a private teacher at our home. It was all about what to expect leading up to and during labor and delivery. We learned how to breathe, how to time contractions, and when to call the doctor. The instructor covered all the topics she felt were necessary and three hours later left us a binder and wished us good luck. Hey, it was better than nothing. If only we had known what we were getting ourselves into by trying to take the easy way out. I learned an important lesson about parenting at this stage: there are no shortcuts. If there is a class your partner wants you to take, listen to her and take it. I wish

THE HEAD SNAP

Speaking of being green to the infant game: I had a few nieces and nephews by this time, so I was somewhat familiar with baby handling. Although I do admit the first time I held my nephew, who was barely three months at the time, his head did that snap-back thing that babies do since their muscle strength has not yet developed. It freaked the hell out of me! I thought it was gonna fall off! Not to mention, I was close to a wall so he could've knocked himself out if he hit it. Way to go, Uncle Chris. I definitely needed a drink after that one. So take it from me, when you pick up your infant, make sure to support baby's neck with your hands at all times. Don't go for the pickup without the support.

someone had told us that when we were at this stage, because in retrospect: I didn't know nuthin'!

Among the benefits of the classroom environment is you can address with other parents all the possible things that can go wrong leading up to and during delivery. Your classmates may come up with questions you would've never thought to ask but are glad to hear the answers to. For instance, knowing how to time the contractions, when to call the doctor, and when to head to the hospital can all seem overwhelming. But once you start dialoguing with other couples about it and chatting with the counselor or doctor on hand, it doesn't seem like such a big deal. Oh, and the good news is that you can head to the hospital anytime. The worst case scenario is that they will send you home if she's not ready.

Another benefit of attending class is the social element. Bonding with other soon-to-be parents and creating a community of support is really helpful, especially for us dads. Parenting makes marriage harder to navigate once the little one comes along. Having friends who are on the same page can make maintaining your new social life with baby doable. Having even one other dad who can give you advice or just shoot the shit with you can bring enormous relief to what can be a stressful adjustment to your new role. Even though my kids are much older, I still make time for a few nights out a month to check in with, hang out with, and bounce issues off my friends and see if there is any great insight they can offer. Or just to drink beer and eat nachos.

At the end of the day, it's all about gathering as much information as possible so you can make the best choices. The choice is yours as to whether you attend classes or not, but as preparation is key, why not start out right? And if you absolutely

---

MARRIAGE COUNSELORS?

True or False: Couples only go to counseling because they are having problems.

Not always true. Many attend to prevent problems, learn to express themselves, and understand each other better before problems come up. You don't have to wait for issues to pile on to seek help. You also don't have to be married to go to a counselor. Just sayin' . . .

---

hate the class you chose, then you can change to another until you find the right fit. It is definitely important to find a comfortable environment so that you can relax and learn.

CHOOSING THE BIRTHING PLACE

Hospital or home: deciding what's best for you.

Who would imagine there are so many choices when it comes to where you can have your baby? Like most clueless men, I just assumed you go to the nearest hospital, or wherever takes your insurance. But once Meredith and I watched some birthing videos in preparation for the big day, I was suddenly aware of a world of choices and options, from hospital to home births.

Reaching out to friends who may have already delivered at various birthing centers is a safe way to weed out places you should avoid. Touring the facility of your choice is also in your best interest. You want to feel comfortable with the setting where she is about to deliver, and for her to be at ease with the environment (well, as at ease as you can be in an environment . . . where she is soon to push a bowling ball through her legs . . .). Eyeing the guest bed and perhaps even sampling it for yourself to see how much sleep you could potentially get is not a bad idea either.

Come prepared with a list of questions. Can you bring your own iPod station? Can you bring your own bedding? And most importantly, can you bring in In-N-Out Burger (or *your* favorite takeout)? Think ahead and ask questions that will help make your experience more relaxed and comfortable.

Getting to know the staff has its benefits too. There were a few nurses that we connected with during my son's birth who made such an impression that we were thrilled they were still around when our second and third kids were born. On the other hand, we made sure we kept our distance from the ones we decided should have chosen a different career path.

You are going to soon discover—if you haven't already—that everyone is going to feel the need to give you advice (warranted or not) about where you should have your kid. There is the passionate group who will insist that home birthing is the *only* way to go. Obviously this is not true. Then there is the equally passionate crowd who feel anything but a hospital is irresponsible. Also not true. Remember, this is your child and the choice is yours.

Bottom line: you want her to have the best pregnancy experience she can possibly have. Ask her these questions: Is she comfortable in a hospital or are there any fears there? Do doctors make her feel more at ease or more stressed? Does the sterile environment make her feel clean or uncomfortable? Can she deal with the drive to the emergency room? Would being at home make her more comfortable or less safe? Who does she want to deliver her baby? If you can open up a dialogue on this subject, you will surely find the best way for her to deliver.

Believe me, I'm no fan of waiting rooms and gurneys. Yet despite my fears of doctors and hospitals, I found it reassuring to know there was a staff of professionals with all sorts of fancy equipment ready to take care of my wife when she was in pain. If you get scared something is going wrong during her pregnancy or the baby arrives prematurely (which is always a shocker, despite knowing it could happen), the emergency room will be a safe haven for the two of you . . . albeit a sterile, slightly terrifying safe haven.

If you opt for a hospital birth, there are a few extra things you can do ahead of time to make the process as smooth as possible. Map out the route to your hospital of choice and figure out the parking situation and who will take care of the kids while you are away (if you already have some).

Also consider having your bags packed ahead of time and in the car as well. When we were having our daughter, Meredith's water broke when we were at home, so we were quite panicked. But Meredith had just packed her bag that night in case of an early delivery (four weeks early for our daughter). Talk about being in touch with your body! It was as if Mer sensed our daughter wasn't gonna stick to the schedule. Unfortunately, being the procrastinator that I am, I did not pack my bag. I was literally throwing random clothes into whatever I could find at the last minute. Good thing there are gift shops at the hospital, as I was forced to buy a toothbrush and toothpaste once I got there.

You should also consider checking into the hospital ahead

of time so you don't have to deal with the paperwork when labor starts. The last thing you need to be doing is fumbling around looking for your insurance card when your wife is doubled over in pain. Ask her obstetrician ahead of time how to do this at the hospital you've selected. Taking care of all the logistics ahead of time makes the experience go much smoother.

THE NAME GAME

How to name your child and avoid names you (and the kid) will regret in the future.

By the time you are seriously thinking of names for your baby, the reality of your situation has hit you like a freight train. It's really happening.

Choosing a name is a personal process. Meredith and I

CAR SEAT A-GO-GO

Hopefully, by the time you and your wife go to the hospital you will have already installed your little one's car seat. If not, you are one badass procrastinator. There are numerous places that can aid in making sure the seat is properly installed, from your local fire department to professional services offered through neighborhood baby stores. Dude, this is one time you don't want to mess around and play Mr. Handyman. If you're not sure you know what to do, have a pro do it for you. Take care of this at least a month before your partner's due date. It's one less thing to think about.

scoured every book we could find to see what name spoke to us. As I mentioned earlier, it's helpful if you begin the search early on, since you may go through numerous changes of heart. The last thing the two of you want is to name your kid something you'll end up regretting.

I recall numerous times growing up when my dad would call me Chrissy instead of Chris. In front of my friends, no less! Talk about humiliating. So when it came time to choose names for our kids, I was particularly sensitive about whether the name would be confusing as to what gender the child was. While one can argue that Kai can be a girl's name as well, it's not the same as being called Chrissy as a boy.

Of course, everyone you know will want to share their ideas as to what name you should choose. Unfortunately it just comes with the territory. If you're lucky, one of your buds will stumble onto something you dig. But mostly it's just the same ol' names you're seeing in your books, or outlandishly bad ideas. "Seven!" demands George Costanza.

There are many traditions that families honor when it comes to naming their child. My brothers and sisters each have at least one child named after a parent. Personally I think that's a bit confusing. Having two people by the same name in one household? On the other hand, I would totally dig naming one of my kids after me.

Keep in mind, the initials of your kid's name are also something to consider. For instance, if your last name is Smith and you name your daughter Allison Sarah, well you can just imagine the embarrassment she will endure when her friends discover her initials are ASS. I on the other hand have to endure the initials CJP. It's funny at first but gets old after a while. I've heard every pee joke in the book.

TERRIBLE, TERRIBLE NAMES

Here's some really awful names I have come across online and in magazines. Shame on their parents. For reals. Look 'em up.

Merle Lester	Mike Litoris
Dick Kock	Allah Magnetic
Oliver Loser	Jed I Knight
DeWanna Boner	Rainbow Aurora
Guy Pinhas	Zuma Rock
Deja Viau	Blanket

As much as we read and searched for a name that spoke to us, it was when we least expected it that the name for our first child hit us on the head. Meredith was talking to a friend one day who mentioned her son's name Kai (short for Chiron). We immediately fell in love with the name Kai. Researching the origin, we found that it meant "ocean" in Hawaiian. As lovers of the ocean, Kai was a no-brainer for us. We later found out that it also means "love and loyalty" in Greek.

Making sure the first name worked with our last name was something we considered as well. My coauthor Frank is unlucky enough to have two hot dog references in his name: Frank (furter) and (Oscar) Meyer. He claims his parents were totally unaware of this. It goes without saying that he has heard every wiener joke known to man.

For us, having a three-syllable last name limited our selection. A single-syllable first name sounded stronger when spoken with our last name. Interestingly a three-syllable name for our daughter worked out quite well too.

Whatever the method you use to choose the name you desire, once you find that name stick with it and don't let anyone change your mind. I love our Kai, Juliette, and Cole. I can't imagine them being named anything different.

BABY SHOWERS AND YOU

What exactly is a baby shower, who is invited, and do you have to go?

Gentlemen, welcome to the new millennium of baby showers, the time-honored bash to honor the mother-to-be and "shower" her with gifts for the bundle-to-be. Traditionally, these gatherings were a female thing: pregnant mamas bonding and noshing with the sacred women in their lives, creating a sort of secret society abounding with obscure games, décor, and sage-like advice from the elders. A society we males had very little notion about. Fast forward to present day, hombres, and suddenly there are ample ways to celebrate the new member of the family, including couples showers involving themes ranging from poker to karaoke to a good old-fashioned BBQ. These days, most folks seem to go the route of inviting couples to the shower. Getting together with the community of friends that mean the most to you is a fun way to share this special event.

My wife and I stuck to the traditional girls-only version, but that was more her friends' doing, as they chose to celebrate their BFF Goddess-style. In fact, despite being half-responsible for the kid to be, I was only allowed to join them at the end as a special janitorial guest employed for my increasingly softening brawn, to shoulder the load of bottles, bibs, pacifiers, stuffed animals, pajamas, towels, robes, books, lullaby CDs, and other gifts. My wife had a marvelous time at the showers for each of our children, bonding with her friends and passing around the new items for all the women to "oooh" and "ahhhh" over as they snacked on cake.

Now, if you are looking to have your own rite of passage with just the guys, then so be it. A friend of mine hosted a dad-chelor party where they went skeet shooting for the afternoon, spewing beers and dirty jokes until they couldn't laugh any harder. Other dudes I know go fishing for the weekend. Maybe a night out at the local pub will do the trick. It's pretty cool to have friends that honor your new role, so if they are down for it, go celebrate.

As far as registering for gifts goes, it would be smart to get a heads up on what you'll need by surfing the Web and registering at stores like Babies "R" Us or Buy Buy Baby. Take a trip with your lady and test-drive the products firsthand. Believe me, it'll be less expensive for you to pay for the party than to pay for all the gear you'll need the first year. Keep in mind that unless someone offers to throw the shower for you, the tab is yours. But that's not so bad when you think about it. After all, you are registering for those necessities you will need once the little one arrives, and then that stuff is given to you free, so you can at least pay for the shower it takes to score it all, right? It's one of the many little side benefits you get along the way . . .

Remember . . .

- The third trimester can be physically and emotionally challenging as the baby's size and position makes it hard for your partner to get comfortable.

- Attend as many classes with her as possible.

- If you want to, you can now find out the sex of your child.

- You could also be thinking about naming your child at this stage.

- If you want a ton of thoughtful baby gifts, get registered and throw yourself a baby shower. Or have a friend or family member do it for you.

CHAPTER

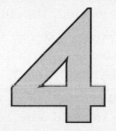

Birth

We talk a lot in this book about staying true to who you are, but one thing to keep in mind is that who you are from this point on will be shaped in part by the experience of your child's birth. Becoming a father opens up your perspective to many things in life, creating a reservoir of love and patience you didn't know existed. Far from detracting from who you are, fatherhood adds to it, embellishes it, and strengthens it. And watching the woman in your life demonstrate levels of strength you previously couldn't fathom definitely helps reinforce the bond between you two.

The birth of your child is hands down the most amazing and surreal thing you will ever experience. Nothing else comes close. When your child takes that first breath, you lose yours. When your child stares into your eyes for the first time, time stops. When those little fingers clutch yours, the earth shifts on its axis. When you first rock your baby to sleep in your arms, you will hardly be able to stand. The number of times you will openly or privately weep is staggering. These are good times, brother. But you do have to be prepared. Especially because the first few days post-birth will be fairly mind-scrambling, and you want to have your act together. Everything is a first for a while. The first time you hold your baby. The first time you feed your child. The first time baby crawls, and so on. Every moment feels significant. And a little terrifying.

But you can make things less terrifying. The more information you can gather, for example, about what your partner will experience during the birth (and what you will see), the better prepared you will be. You need to keep your act together during this mind-blowing event, so make sure you know what's coming (or simply read on, intrepid dad-to-be). You should also be making decisions on who gets to visit in the hospital room after she delivers, if she wants an epidural, if you want to cut the cord, and if you want to go the circumcision route if you have a boy. These are decisions you do not want to make on the fly, dude, and do not want to make alone. Obviously all of these need to be decided ahead of time.

HOW DO YOU KNOW IT'S TIME?

The calm before the storm . . .

My coauthor Frank told me a story about his ex-wife's water breaking. She was midway through cooking up a pot of home-made chili when she felt a strange sensation and looked down to see the kitchen floor covered in water. He worked an hour away, so she jumped in the car and drove herself to the hospital, calling Frank to meet her there as she raced out the door. Her delivery lasted over thirty hours, and at some point when Frank offered to run home and grab her some stuff she wanted by her side, she mentioned, "Oh, there's chili in the fridge if you're hungry." But how was that possible since her water broke halfway through making it and she had to dash off to the hospital? "Well, I finished making the chili first!" That, dudes, is a strong woman! They call that recipe Bella Chili after their daughter, by the way.

As you get closer to her delivery date (and remember that many first-time moms deliver up to two weeks early), you'll want to have bags packed, a hospital room booked, a route all mapped out, and be ready to head to the hospital at a moment's notice.

How do you know it's time to go to the hospital? Every labor

➤ THE LAST MEALS

My wife's last dinner before she delivered our first child was a grilled cheese sandwich and fries with a chocolate milkshake at a fifties dinner in LA. However, many feel that spicy food is the way to go at this stage, especially if you are late in delivery. An old wives' tale claims that spicy foods induce labor, so this might be the time to order in a curry dish from your favorite Indian or Moroccan restaurant. There's even a restaurant in LA famous for a spicy salad that is said to induce labor for overdue pregnant women. Some women swear by it!

is different. Discuss with your doctor ahead of time when you should be ready to go. And if your partner thinks labor is starting and/or you have any questions, call your doctor. He or she can advise you on next best steps. The answer will depend on a variety of factors, from whether or not your partner's water has broken (a sign your baby is ready to come) to the frequency and duration of contractions (usually a duration of forty-five to sixty seconds, occurring five minutes apart). If you are at all uncertain or your partner is in extreme pain, call your doctor.

GETTING TO KNOW YOUR HOSPITAL

Booking a room and preparing for the birth.

Keep in mind, it can be a long time from the moment she begins labor to the actual delivery. Labor can last anywhere from a few hours to a day or more, but a typical first-time mother usually takes eight to fourteen hours. Labor occurs in three stages: early/active labor, delivery of baby, and delivery of placenta. How long labor lasts and how it progresses is different for every woman. Regardless, you'll want to get to know your hospital before your child arrives.

Depending on the place and space available, you may be transitioning from predelivery to delivery to a postpartum room once your baby is born. Some hospitals have private rooms available, while at others the rooms are shared. Depending on your insurance plan and availability, you may be able to score a private room. Either way, you will learn more when you take a tour of your local facility.

Until the delivery, your partner will probably spend a lot of time in a predelivery room, where they monitor her until she is ready to deliver. Once her cervix is fully dilated, the second stage of labor begins: the final descent and birth of your baby. That's when she will be moved into the actual delivery room (unless your hospital does all this in one room, which some do). At the beginning of the second stage, her contractions might be a little farther apart, giving her (and you!) a chance to get some rest before the real work begins.

Once your partner is ten centimeters dilated (about the size of a baby's head,) baby is almost here. Until then, settle into your new digs, scope out the joint for food, coffee stations, etc. There is likely to be a bathroom available in the predelivery room, but be smart. If you have to unload, so to speak, use a bathroom in the hallway. In her highly sensitive state, with her antenna up as high as it can go, you do not need to fill her cramped room with your funky back-door odor.

Make the transition to hospital life much more comfortable by bringing items from your home with you. Whether it's your pillow, comforter, sheets, pictures, or music, make sure you decide ahead of time and plan it out. Your iPhone can be your best friend during this time, so make sure you remember your carrying case and/or your charger.

> **GET A ROOM!**

You can book a postpartum room for your partner to stay in for a few days while she recuperates. This is especially wise if your lady has a C-section, as she'll need some extra time to get back on her feet.

Chances are, your lady won't be eating much while in labor. If it's just the two of you, you'll be by her side most of the time distracting her from her pain, so there's not much time for a food run. But if you allow others to join and support you, you may be fortunate enough to find a free moment to hit the vending machine for a snack or coffee. Just don't go too far. You don't want to miss any action. My sister has still never forgiven my dad for not making it to the delivery room when she was born. Apparently he went to make a phone call, and when he came back, she was already there. Don't let that be you.

YOUR ROLE DURING LABOR

What you can do while she is doing the heavy lifting.

The active labor process is unpredictable: you don't know how long it will last or how much pain your partner will endure. But one thing you can control is how the two of you will get along. This, my friend, will depend mostly on you. No pressure, right?

From this point on, you are in charge of one thing and one thing only: making your partner your first priority. You are her cheerleader, her advocate, her voice of reason, her therapist, and her waiter. You name it, that's you. Be prepared for moments of irritability and exhaustion on her part. Most of all, do not to take it personally if your partner makes comments that offend or upset you. And be sure you don't do the same. Now is not the time to pick a fight or even fire back if a shot comes across your bow. Your partner has an excuse; you don't.

> **DID YOU KNOW?**
>
> Once she reaches thirty-seven weeks, she is considered to be at full term of her pregnancy, though delivery may not actually happen for a few more weeks.

Oh, and if you are a jokester, this may not be the time to try to lighten the mood with your randy Howard Stern–influenced comedy chops.

There will be a lot of waiting around during the next day or so. Patience is your best friend during this phase, and distraction will be the necessary tool that saves you from getting into trouble. It would be smart to discuss ahead of time with your partner some ways to pass the time while she is in labor. Consider a favorite movie you guys can watch in your room or visits from close friends to help distract you both. Whatever you decide, it's good to have a plan.

One thing's for certain: during your partner's labor, you'll be shouldering a big load of responsibility, and if you are smart, you will graciously accept help from extras. Your better half will probably want some extra crew on board for support too. After all, she will be doing all the heavy lifting, so to speak, so give her whatever she needs to be comfortable.

For our first child's birth it was almost like a party. Meredith has a pretty tight-knit group of gals who were all over at our place enjoying dinner and watching some mindless TV. When her contractions got way out of hand we all hightailed it to the hospital convoy-style. Her friends turned out to be a reliable distraction from the increasing pain she was in as her contractions began to go crazy, keeping her attention on silly childhood stories, walks down the halls, and bathroom trips. Yes, even then they went together. Her mom was part of the posse that participated in calming her nerves and reminding her how to breathe and relax. I was thrilled to have the assistance.

Delivery is an exhausting experience. Trust me, there were numerous times when Meredith was getting annoyed with me. That was my cue to hang back and let her gals take over. Don't take it personally, as your partner is being flooded with all sorts of feelings and emotions. In fact, she may say some things to you that she will regret. One friend told me his wife cried out during delivery that she hated him for getting her pregnant. Now *that's* a pretty strong statement. She didn't even remember saying that to him when he brought it up afterward.

But what if the pain is too much for her, you wonder? Well, they have some remedies for that, and the most popular one is epidural anesthesia. An epidural is local anesthesia that blocks pain in a specific area of the body. The goal is to provide regional pain relief, as opposed to straight-up anesthesia, which leads to total lack of feeling. Epidurals block the nerve impulses from the lower spinal segments, resulting in reduced sensation in the lower half of the body.

When is the best time to get an epidural? You want her to be in active labor before starting the process, which means waiting until she's about four or five centimeters dilated with regular contractions (the fear is that the epidural might slow down her contractions). It's never too late to get an epidural, unless the baby's head is crowning, so if you get to the hospital before she's actually in active labor, you can ask the anesthesiologist to place the catheter as soon as you're settled in your bed. Then you can wait to start the medication until your labor becomes active. But once baby's head is crowning (or if the doctor feels your partner will not be able to sit still for the procedure), Mom will lose her opportunity and have to suffer through any pain.

Many women opt out of epidurals since they do not like the idea of drugs potentially affecting their baby or causing other side effects. The choice is yours, and researching the pros and cons ahead of time is smart. It goes without saying that understanding the different types of epidurals, how they are administered, and their risks and benefits, will help with the decision-making process during labor. Again, having a plan will reduce your stress and hopefully make your experience more enjoyable.

There are many different ways the delivery can go for her, from quick and easy (well, easy is a relative term here) to long and torturous. Each of our children's deliveries was totally different.

Our first was pretty much by the book: the long, drawn out labor period, the intense pushing for hours, and finally the moment I saw my son's head for the first time. Once he was delivered, I was shocked to hear what the doctor said next: "Okay, get ready for part two." Part two? What the hell was he talking about? He was talking about the delivery of the placenta. Just like the baby, the placenta needs to be pushed out as well. This is where you need to either get over your squeamishness about blood or excuse yourself from the room.

For our second child, Juliette, Meredith ended up delivering four weeks early. Ironically, the night before, Meredith and I decided to watch the video of Kai's birth. It was as if Juliette wanted to come and meet Kai as soon as possible because it was early the next morning that Meredith was woken up by what she thought was the need to pee. It turned out that her water broke and we hauled ass to the hospital. Once we arrived, Meredith was taken to a delivery room where they monitored her. We calmed down for a spell. Hey, we had done this before, right? What could go wrong this time? Suddenly a team in yellow hazmat suits stormed in and for a second it seemed like all hell had broken loose in the panic zone! Turns out, it was simply the vacuum crew, who sometimes lend a hand in the delivery process. They apologized for the scare and split. Whew!

For our Cole, we needed an emergency delivery since he was seven and a half weeks early. Since the baby was arriving so fast and unexpectedly, Meredith was forbidden by the doctors from choosing an epidural even if she wanted one. I've never seen anyone handle so much pain with such power and composure. Luckily there were no complications, and our son was born healthy and strong. Granted, he did have to live in the NICU for three and a half weeks but fortunately, with the best of care, he continued to mature and grow.

STAYING SANE

Keeping your head together as you stand on the brink of a new world. What you can do to help as she delivers.

Let me be clear about this: there is no way to stay sane during delivery. All the homework and prep you can do is not the same as actually experiencing it. You are still going to end up making mistakes, things will go wrong, fights will erupt, or you will simply get a fear in the pit of your stomach that seems unshakable. That's just part of life in general, dude, especially in the face of stress. You have to be flexible during this whole experience. The more knowledge you can have, the better, but also use your instincts and go with your gut.

One word you often don't hear used to describe labor is *tedious*. It's true though. Between all the exciting and scary moments, and the contractions and shrieking pain, there are long stretches of boredom. And she's really uncomfortable. So help take your wife's mind off her discomfort by keeping her busy. Keep her occupied with music, conversation, and card games. In my case, my wife's friends helped tremendously with this, but be ready to get into the mix!

Get approval from your partner before you post updates from the hospital with photos on Facebook, Twitter, or Instagram. Stick to simple status posts on her condition to keep your friends updated, and be easy with the photos. She's probably not going to feel very confident about her appearance, so don't go broadcasting her to the world.

Once she gets hooked up to the monitor and is restricted to the bed, focus on ways to get your partner to relax. Rub her feet, arms, legs, back, and neck. If you brought some aromatherapy oils and soothing music, now would be a good time to get those going. Turn your phone on vibrate so you don't have any distractions. Try to create a calm atmosphere for your baby's arrival.

From this point on, your partner will be closely monitored, but that doesn't mean you can't step in for help. Doctors and nurses will be coming in and out sporadically, but if your partner feels that the time is now and this baby is coming, you better hightail it out the door for some assistance.

THE BABY'S HERE!

Cutting the cord, meconium, and sights you will never forget!

Depending on your personality, being thoroughly freaked out as a parent may start from the moment your baby is born. For instance, there will be blood. If you are disturbed by blood, then you need to come up with a plan to survive delivery. I know some dudes who actually fainted. If you even think this is a possibility, then you better address it with your partner ahead of time. If you have no idea, then it may serve you to watch a few birthing videos to test your tolerance.

Another thing you need to be warned about is something your partner will be horrified to discuss, but I'm gonna let you in on it. Poo poo. Yes, during the delivery process it is possible that you partner can actually . . . er . . . "drop a kid off at the pool" while she is pushing the baby out. While I have never witnessed this act myself, it is good to wrap your head around the concept so it doesn't completely blow your mind if it happens. This is completely natural and virtually impossible to control. Most likely your partner will not even know it is happening, so if she asks, I would advise staying cool and acting as if you have no idea what she is talking about. It's one of those little white lies that everyone appreciates.

If your partner is experiencing labor for a particularly long time, it is possible the doctor may suggest Pitocin, a synthetic form of a naturally occurring hormone called oxytocin, to speed up the process. This will be administered through an IV. It would be smart to ask your partner how she feels about the possibility ahead of time so that if it comes to this choice, she can make an informed decision. Your partner will not be in the best mind-set to do this if she has been experiencing labor for a long period of time. Remember, you are trying to reduce her stress, not increase it.

In the midst of all of this, your baby will arrive. I'm telling you now: nothing I say here can prepare you for the feeling that overwhelms you once you first lay eyes on your baby. Even the toughest dudes I know have shed a tear when they caught their first glimpse of their newborn. And once you actually hold your child in your arms? At that moment, all of life's distractions go out the window. It's amazing how someone so small can create a feeling so big.

Once out, your child will not yet be able to regulate his or her temperature so the nurse will wrap baby in a blanket to keep warm. Immediately the staff will use suction to clear baby's passages of the amniotic fluid ingested while in your partner's womb. A series of tests will occur (also known as an Apgar assessment) to confirm that your baby is healthy. The tests include evaluating your baby's heart rate, breathing, muscle tone, reflex response, and color. Next the umbilical cord will be cut. A clamp is paced on the cord in preparation. After the cord is cut, some blood is immediately taken from it to determine your child's blood type. A little stump remains, and they put a clamp on it.

Seeing your baby with what looks like a plastic clothespin on the belly button is a bit painful to view. Thankfully, it doesn't hurt your child. But it always gave me the shivers when it came time to clean the stump. Eventually it gets all brown and hard like a big-ass scab, and eventually it falls off. Some people keep it as a memento. I know someone who made a necklace out of her child's belly stump. I love my kids, but for me, that's an extreme token of devotion there.

Speaking of dark brown stuff, your baby's poop is going to be just that. Now would be a good time to familiarize yourself with the term *meconium*. Meconium resembles sticky tar and is composed of the contents your baby ingests while in the womb. If you don't know this ahead of time, believe me, you'll soon be asking your doctor what the hell is going on. Don't worry, it eventually runs its course once your baby starts drinking milk. If your partner breast-feeds, then the poop turns a grainy yellow color. That's normal too. How fun to learn so much about your baby's shit, right? Oh, the joys of parenting.

THE ABCS OF C-SECTIONS

Some women might need to undergo a Cesarean birth.
Man up . . . it can be tough . . .

There is always a slim chance that during the labor process an emergency C-section will be performed—that is, if the baby is breech (butt first as opposed to head) or due to placenta previa (a condition where the placenta covers the cervix and blocks the delivery channel between the uterus and vagina). In this case, the feeling of helplessness may soon set in. How do you prepare? What do you do?

Even though you may be overwhelmed, fearful, or stressed, your survival skills will kick in. All the preparation you've done up to this point will take over, and you need to trust it, along

> ⟶ **POSTPARTUM BLEEDING**
>
> Some women may bleed quite a bit after birth. Don't let this freak you out at first. This could be a normal variation from delivery. If the bleeding continues for an extended period of time, then she needs to follow up with her doctor. She should also change pads throughout the day, so don't keep asking why she's off to the bathroom yet again. Some nurses even give out numbing spray for her to spritz on her privates, or even maxi pad–shaped ice packs to place inside the disposable mesh underwear.

with the doctors and nurses. It's your job to be calm and follow their orders.

In a Cesarean birth, there will be a sterile sheet that is used to separate the lower half of your partner from your view. During the operation you will assist your partner by sitting next to her head, holding her hand, and keeping her comfortable. Once your baby is delivered, you can look over the sheet to catch your first glimpse of your baby as the doctor hands him off to the nurse. She will perform some tasks, like suctioning, warming, and cleaning your infant. Once those are completed, baby will be handed over for you to take over. Your partner will experience another thirty minutes or so of the doctor sewing up the incision used for delivery. Most times, your baby can get a few minutes of time with Mom to bond, but once that is over I would suggest you shadow the nurse and continue your bonding process. However, in emergency situations you may need to wait in the waiting room as opposed to being by your partner's side.

Depending on the size of your child, your partner's doctor may need to perform something called an episiotomy. This is the process of making a small incision in the perineum (the small space between the vaginal opening and the anus) to make delivery easier and reduce the risk of tearing occurring, which can be both painful and difficult to repair. Shortly after birth the cut is repaired with sutures. If you have a hard time with blood, it's good to have knowledge of these procedures so you are prepared. Things happen fast during the delivery process once it gets moving. Ask your doctor about these options and situations so you can be educated and prepared. Knowledge is ammunition.

My hope is that you will never need to encounter the intensity of emergency situations. However, because you are a parent, they are practically unavoidable. How you handle these situations will determine how successfully you come out of them. So use the time beforehand to educate yourself for any possible scenario, then let it go. If needed, your instincts will kick in and you will know what to do. That's parenting in a nutshell.

Speaking of the joys of parenting . . .

TO CUT OR NOT TO CUT
The raging circumcision debate.

Circumcision is a topic that spurs a great deal of controversy. Why is this such a heated issue? In Santa Monica, California, there was a proposal to ban circumcisions entirely. Recently,

> **DID YOU KNOW?**
>
> Circumcision was once believed to be a cure for paralysis. Yup, in the late 1800s doctors turned to circumcision to "cure" a variety of ailments, from paralysis to fevers to brass poisoning. It wasn't until 1870 that the medical community could wrap its collective head around circumcision and cut away the nonsense (bad pun, sorry). The current popular belief is that circumcised boys are less likely to develop urinary tract infections than noncircumcised boys. Plus, they have a little less cleaning to do in that area than the non-chop-tops.

San Francisco anti-circumcision activists gathered enough signatures to place the issue on the ballot. They were looking to pass a law that would result in a $1,000 fine and up to a year in jail if a circumcision was performed. The initiative was dropped as it was ruled that only a state could regulate medical procedures. Fortunately (or unfortunately, depending on your stance) the new statewide law in California prevents further efforts to ban circumcisions by cities or counties. But if enough people were inspired by this issue to put a ban on the ballot, then you know we are talking about a heated, passionate subject.

People wonder if being circumcised leaves some sort of mental scar on a boy, a horrifying image that will haunt him later in life. At the risk of giving too much information, I'm just gonna admit that, yes, I was circumcised as a baby. Let me confirm that I DO NOT REMEMBER IT ONE BIT! I do not have any flashbacks, nightmares, sudden inexplicable pain between my legs, or fear of knives or doctors.

That being said, I will freely admit that seeing my boy get circumcised was the single most disturbing event I have ever witnessed.

The question of circumcision is for you and your baby momma to decide and no one else. If you are not religious, then perhaps this is not an issue. If you don't see the possible hygiene risks as important, then you may not need to think twice. And if you are not happy with the decision your folks made for your body, then here's a chance to do the right thing with your boy.

I would highly suggest weighing your options and discussing the pros and cons before making your final decision. The last thing you want to do it is leave it up to your kid to decide when he is an adult. Oooooh, I just got a horrible pain between my legs when I wrote that. Bottom line: this is a decision you cannot avoid . . . unless of course you have a girl.

BABY PARANOIA

What if they misplace our baby? Who will protect it? And who will protect them from me if they lose my friggin' kid?!?

I can still see that pained look on Kai's face and hear his roar as the doctor lifted him up and announced his arrival. It was as if he was pissed we had taken him out of his warm, comfortable nest and he wanted to go back.

The moment Kai arrived, I was both elated and freaked out. Being handed scissors and asked to cut the cord by the doctor was something I had not considered ahead of time. You want ME to cut THAT thing?!?! It was more than a bit disturb-

> ### ➤ WHAT'S THAT STUFF?
>
> The white, creamy biofilm covering the skin of the fetus during the last trimester of pregnancy, Vernix caseosa is a naturally occurring coating on the neonatal skin that helps protect it.

ing, and I can still feel the sensation of the scissors cutting through. The cord was thicker than I thought, and it took some effort to get the job done. I was creeped out thinking I could be hurting this tiny, helpless baby, not to mention Meredith. I recently learned that the umbilical cord doesn't have pain-sensitive nerve fibers, so cutting it doesn't hurt the baby or Mom. NOW I find this out?

Watching the nurses handle Kai once he was born was a trip: flipping him over like he was a pancake, scrubbing off the Vernix caseosa (that white cottage cheese stuff around baby's skin) covering his body, not to mention sticking that unusually large nasal aspirator up his nose and down his throat to remove the excess liquid from the amniotic fluid. I wanted to jump in and shout, "Not so rough or you'll break him!" Later I learned it is the nurses' experience and confidence that allows them to be so nonchalant. They can handle that stuff in their sleep. Thankfully, they were awake for Kai.

Once he was cleaned up, our nurse wrapped Kai in a blanket so tight I thought he was going to suffocate. This is what they call swaddling. Essentially your kid looks like a burrito once this process is properly executed. There is an art to doing this, and believe it or not, your child actually likes it. (By the

> ## ───► BURRITO TIME!
>
> Whether you enjoy a tasty burrito or not, there are many good reasons to wrap your baby tightly in the form of one:
>
> - Swaddling regulates baby's body temperature.
>
> - It reduces the chance that the startle reflex will wake the sleeping giant.
>
> - Helps the li'l one to feel more safe and secure during those first three to four months.
>
> - Reduces crying in infants, especially babies with colic or acid reflux.
>
> - Swaddling helps babies get the sleep they need during this developmental stage.

way, try to take as many of the blankets and beanies they give you at the hospital as possible to use when you get home. It'll save you buying them later on, and they can double as burp cloths too. Much later you can use them as rags to wash your car and sop up spilled beer!)

There will be so much to take in once your little one is born, so try to breathe easy and stay calm. Meredith was paranoid that he could accidently get switched with another kid in the hospital, so she was adamant that I go with our nurse to the nursery and watch him get tagged with his ID bracelet. Okay, maybe she had watched one too many Lifetime movies during her pregnancy, but I have to admit that the same thought had crossed my mind, so I was stoked she had me tag along. I made sure I was on top of where my little burrito was going and what was being done to him at all times. It made Meredith feel more secure, and I was happy to ease her anxiety. My baby stalker tendencies did create a bit of tension with the nursing staff, but at the end of the day I go home to my wife not the nurse, so be smart and do the same if your partner requests it.

Once Kai was settled and brought back to our room, we were left to fend for ourselves. I can still see him lying in the clear plastic bin they gave us (at an angle so he was not lying on his back, which keeps him from swallowing or choking on the amniotic fluid still inside). I was so wiped out at this point that all I wanted to do was sleep. The problem was that I couldn't. Every time Kai made a noise, I would leap out of my chair to check and see if he was choking and to be sure he was still breathing. I was in shock that we were left to take care of him alone at this point. What the hell did we know? No one came in to check on us for hours. For our later children, that was not a problem since we were already seasoned parents. But

---

PUSH GIFTS

Many guys buy a gift for their spouse after she gives birth. Ironically, they call it a "push gift," which I find to be hilarious. It may seem a little petty ("Hey, you just had my child, here's a stuffed unicorn!"), but it's a nice thought and shows you are thinking of her. Hospitals have gift shops, and I suggest you use them.

this was our first, so how would they know if we had any idea what we were doing? It's something to think about when you are deciding whether to have your baby sleep in the nursery the first few nights or in your room. Both are completely acceptable; this is a decision that needs to be made based on your comfort level, but if I were to do it again I might choose to let my firstborn be taken care of by the nurses so we could tend to ourselves for a bit in our little white room.

THE LITTLE WHITE ROOM

You'll be spending a lot of time in the hospital over the next few days, so make the best of it and be useful.

So the baby has arrived and now you two are living out of her hospital room for the next few days. Make the best of it, dude, and be helpful. Your days in the hospital will feel like a whirlwind, as information will be hurtling at you from every direction, so I suggest you keep your eyes and ears open. Maybe even bring a pen and pad to take notes. Better yet, if you have a smart phone, use the voice memo app to make it easier on yourself. There will be numerous lessons to learn, like how to give your little one a bath, how to clean the umbilical cord, and how to clean out baby's nose. Meredith was so exhausted after Kai was born that she barely had the energy to learn how to breast-feed him. This is where I stepped in and where you can too. There was a lactation specialist on staff who educated us on techniques for successful breast-feeding. She even called one of the methods for cradling the baby the "football

➤ **BABY ON BOARD**

If you plan on driving Mom and baby home after the hospital, you are going to need an appropriate child restraint fitted. Infant seats are normally for babies that weigh approximately twenty-two pounds or less and are twenty-five inches or less in length. Every single time an infant or child rides in a car, he or she needs to be protected by the appropriate child restraints (not the adult safety belt alone). Children can be seriously injured or strangled if the shoulder belt gets wrapped around their neck. Most people know this, but the seat/restraint should not be used in the front seat of the vehicle. And never hold your baby in your arms while riding in a vehicle.

hold," which I was able to relate to immediately. Holding Kai like a running back racing down the field with a football gripped to his side was practically the only way to get him to respond and eat.

Meredith appreciated my enthusiasm and newly gained knowledge and was thankful I had been paying attention since the hospital was too overstimulating at that time for her to remember much.

You'll probably be presented with the opportunity to have your baby's photo taken in the hospital for a nominal fee, but since every phone has a camera these days, you can do it yourself and save some dough. But be sure to fill out the information correctly when completing the birth certificate. I would also strongly advise ordering a few extra copies to keep on hand. Believe it or not, you will need extras when your kids get older. My kids need to provide proof of age for baseball, and an original birth certificate is mandatory. Handing over baby's original birth certificate would suck, so I'm happy I have extras. Be sure to store them in a fireproof place. But don't be like me and forget where you put them!

Once home, we eventually acclimated to our new lifestyle and slowly found our rhythm. The transition is a bit startling at first, but once you get your baby on a schedule, you will find life and baby soon calm down.

Remember . . .

- Time to find your birthing place. Go check out the hospitals or alternatives near you, take a tour, pick or confirm your doctor, reserve a room, and look at the food options on hand.

- Start thinking about who you want to be at the hospital when she gives birth. This can get political, so be careful.

- While it's unlikely someone is going to lose or steal your baby, it's normal to feel a little paranoia about this.

- Things can get tense and scary during labor. Water breaking, blood, meconium, and cutting the cord are just some of the things that could gross you out during the labor process. Set a good example and don't freak out.

- Whatever your stance is on circumcision, you want to have made your decision by now.

CHAPTER

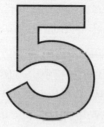

Life with Baby

Dude, nine months ago you probably felt like you would never get to this day, but you made it. Congratulations!

But the real adventure is just beginning. Now that there are three (or more) of you in the picture, not only will you be managing your new role as dad, but you still have your other role as a [insert your professional occupation here], not to mention that of husband too. Think of these past nine months as the hazing period. In fact, you'll probably literally feel like you are in a haze from the lack of sleep, but that just comes along with the territory.

Pre-children, I used to view life as challenging and over-whelming, as I juggled work, pursuing goals, exercise, etc. It felt like there was never enough time in the day to get things done. Now I look back and wonder what the hell I was thinking.

Life was so much simpler back then, so carefree. That being said, I wouldn't trade my current life as a father of three for any of that. My life then wasn't nearly as fulfilling as my life is now. But I didn't know that until I experienced what it was like to have a child. No matter how much you read in books or watch on TV, nothing is going to prepare you more for being a dad than experiencing it for yourself.

In the months after your child's birth, you and your partner will figure out a routine that works, and before you know it you'll be taking on the mantle of father without a second thought. At first, though, it's going to seem strange. Think of it like starting a new job. It takes time to fit into a new environment, to get into a new groove. The first few weeks are a bit rough since you don't know what to expect. I can almost guarantee that you will be up numerous times throughout the night, but thankfully you can catch some Zs during the day if your work schedule permits. If you are lucky enough to have taken a week or two off from work once your baby was born, than you can use the day to catch up on much needed rest. Eventually your body will get used to the new schedule and you'll figure out a way to make it work. For the first few months, though, the best thing you can do is to be open to whatever is thrown your way. Consider yourself in training mode.

During this time, a lot of the work is going to be shouldered by your partner, especially if she chooses to breast-feed. But that's okay—you can still help. Whether it's a diaper change, a bottle feeding, or soothing your little one to sleep, being available to assist in every way you can is going to make the transition much easier for everyone.

BRINGING HOME BABY

A chat about postpartum depression, dealing with friends and relatives, some clothing, baby food, and baby gear recommendations, and an overview of what lies ahead.

For months before his arrival, I would stroll into Kai's room, plop down on the floor, and dream about what it was going to be like to be a dad. Of course, my thoughts were of the two of us throwing a baseball, surfing in the ocean, getting him on a bike for the first time, walking the dog . . . you know, your typical dad experiences.

After he arrived, when I fell into that daydream, I was usually awakened by the shrill of Kai's powerful pipes. I was a slave to feedings, changings, and the loving gaze my loud child bestowed upon me, but when it got tough, I reminded myself that there is no feeling in the world quite like the tiny grip of your child's hand as his little fingers squeeze yours.

For the most part, the first few weeks will entail your child

---

➤ FREEZING BREAST MILK

Many women freeze their breast milk to use for later. This is especially useful if she is using the pump, because sometimes once they get started those breasts don't wanna quit! While it may be creepy for us dudes to open a freezer full of tiny bottles of breast milk, it's a way better alternative than a screaming baby and a sore, angry mommy. And pumping may help give her boobs a much-needed break.

feeding, sleeping, and pooping. I encourage you to split these responsibilities, so your partner won't feel alone during this new stage and you can experience bonding with your new baby. Since all my kids were breast-fed, I didn't have that much to do in regards to feedings. But I did help out when it came time for burping, changing diapers, and putting them to sleep.

Don't freak out when you discover your newborn losing weight when he or she first comes home from the hospital. It's actually typical for your baby to lose about 7 percent of body weight after birth, but your doctor will help you monitor this so you can make sure your little one is healthy.

It's recommended you feed your baby every two hours in order to get that weight back to normal by the first doctor visit two weeks later. So if you break that down by twenty-four hours, you are looking at twelve feedings per day. That's a lot of work on your partner's part, so any opportunity for you to help out will be welcomed. Diaper changes should amount to at least four in a twenty-four-hour period, although from what I can recall, I pretty much ended up changing diapers after every feeding. That's a lot of poop, right?

FORMULA FACTS

It's easy to overfeed when using formula because it takes less effort for baby to drink from a bottle than from a breast. Best to make sure the nipple hole on the bottle is the right size so the liquid can drip slowly and not pour out. Also, if baby shows signs of being full before the bottle is empty, don't feel the need to finish off the bottle. You don't want to overfeed.

Give your partner a chance to recuperate from the feedings. If she is at all stressed out or too tired, it will make it more challenging for her to produce milk, which will in turn make your baby more frustrated that he or she can't eat as easily, and that will make you feel helpless too. See the chain effect happening here? You and your partner should also do your best to help each other catch up on sleep whenever possible, because with your little one, it's pretty much a given that you won't be sleeping as much as you will need or want to.

Taking constant care of a newborn, chances are your partner is going to get cabin fever pretty quick. Sometimes it's a challenge for moms to adjust to this new life, especially if they have been pretty active pre-pregnancy working full-time or via other commitments. Granted, of all the moms I've interviewed, none ever regretted having children, but several did experience postpartum depression due to the change in hormones

→ BABY BLUES

Many new mothers experience mood swings and crying spells after childbirth, but some face a more intense, long-lasting form of depression. This is postpartum depression. They call it the baby blues, but it is much more serious then that cutesy moniker implies. Postpartum depression isn't a character flaw or a weakness. You can try to talk rationally with your partner about it, but she just can't get out of that funk and nothing you say will help. If you sense that your partner is depressed, talk to your doctor and seek treatment, so you both can enjoy your baby and this new phase of your life.

and lack of interaction with the outside world. If you're concerned that she has postpartum depression, talk to your doctor right away.

Dude, you need to be supportive of your wife during this time. Don't try to solve your partner's problems, but lend an ear to show support. And once you're comfortable enough to leave baby with a trusted family member or friend, a date night could also help. Get her back out in the world and feeling like a human being again.

After Kai was born, there were days when Meredith and I would head out for a walk with him in the stroller. That was a fine way to feel connected to the rest of the world and to combat feeling like homebodies. In fact, taking your child outside to see the world and smile at passersby can be terrific for baby as well as the two of you. There's no reason your child should be sequestered. You'll probably be feeling super-protective at this early stage, but it's healthy and productive for your child to start interacting with the outside world.

For a first-time parent, or even an experienced parent, my philosophy is *better safe than sorry*. So if you are unclear about a certain situation in these first weeks at home, like if your baby seems to be crying unusually long or is not eating as much, call the doctor. In the beginning you may feel like you are calling about every little thing, but eventually your confidence will grow and you will be able to handle whatever is thrown your way. The doctor is there for a reason—to help. Take advantage of this.

BABY-PROOFING

Getting your home ready for the oncoming tornado that is your little one.

To this day, there is one drawer in our kitchen that I keep forgetting is baby-proofed. We're talking thirteen years later and I still can't remember! As much of a pain as baby-proofing can be, it is something you need to do or at least consider. For the first few months, you will not need to worry about your little one getting into anything since baby will not yet be mobile. But once they start moving, forget about it. Babies manage to get themselves into everything and anything.

There are many ways to go about baby-proofing your home. Some parents use professional services that will come in and set you up from top to bottom, although it can cost you a pretty penny. The more common option is to just do it yourself. But how?

When beginning to baby-proof your home, get down on all fours in order to get a firsthand view of your home from your child's perspective. By crawling around on the floor, you will be able to see those sharp edges or dangling wires that can pose a danger to your little munchkin. It goes without saying that if you poke your eye out during this experiment then you've discovered something that needs to be removed or baby-proofed (and you may have to see a doctor about that eye). Be sure to pull on end tables and bookcases to see how sturdy they are, and to see what items on top can easily fall off. Once your little one begins to stand, he or she is going to need some assistance, and if you are not around, you can bet your ass that bookcase is going to replace you. Make sure you bolt

4 WAYS TO PROTECT YOUR BABY

Here are the four big threats to your baby around your house:

- **Choking and Suffocation:** Avoid toys with eyes, buttons, or other pieces that baby can pull off and swallow. Don't sleep with your infant, as you can roll over and squash 'em. Put baby down on his or her back to sleep.

- **Falling:** According to the CDC (Centers for Disease Control and Prevention), falling is the leading cause of nonfatal injury to babies under twelve months. Over 100,000 infants are hurt every year from this! Yikes! Keep an eye on where your baby is, and monitor situations closely to avoid tumbles.

- **Burns:** Burns are the fourth-leading cause of accidental deaths and injuries to infants, so don't carry hot food or drinks or use the stove while holding the baby. Always unplug and put away blow-dryers and irons after each use. Set your hot-water heater to no more than 120 degrees to prevent the chance of scalding.

- **Poison:** No, not the eighties band! I'm talking about dangerous household items us adults know not to swallow. The smallest amount of a poisonous substance can hit the baby hard because baby's so small, has a fast metabolism, and has low defenses against toxins. So lock all cabinets and drawers that contain cleaning products, medications, and other toxic stuff. Post the National Capital Poison Control Center's number (800-222-1222) on your fridge.

You should also be aware that houses built before 1978 can contain lead paint, which can be dangerous. To decrease your family's exposure to lead, have your home tested by a professional and fix any hazards you're made aware of. If there is even a slight fear of this, then have your doctor administer a blood test on your child, as this can detect high levels of lead.

big-ticket items like these to the wall to ensure your child's safety.

Today there are a slew of alternatives to conventional baby-proofing. Some people use their rubber bracelets to clamp cabinet doors together instead of buying plastic clasps, or use PVC piping to build a homemade gate to keep baby confined to one area of the house. If you employ any of these methods, make sure you test them carefully to make sure they'll withstand baby's curious hands. Another example: you can make your own corner cushions by cutting a tennis ball in half and securing it over the edge of a sharp-ended coffee table. Of course, it my not be the most attractive décor for your house and might tarnish your feng shui, but once your kid comes along it's going to be pretty chaotic. Maintaining cool appearances will be the least of your worries for a little while.

Babies are drawn to electrical outlets like magnets. So after you've given your pad a baby-view once-over, do an outlet sweep and cover 'em all with those little plastic protectors. While you're at it, make sure you choose outlet covers that are safe. Some out there on the market can be a choking hazard if your little one is talented enough to get them off (and speaking from experience, I can almost guarantee that will happen).

These days, there are a variety of eco-friendly cleaning supplies on the market. Since your baby will occupy most of the time lying and crawling on the floor, you will want to make sure the materials used to keep the floor clean are safe. Check out brands like Method or Seventh Generation. If you are really ambitious, you can Google some cleaning solutions simply made from lemons, vinegar, and water. Aromatherapy oils like tea tree and eucalyptus can also be possible options. But be sure to keep these high on the shelf, away from your baby's reach.

You don't want your child to feel trapped like a caged beast, but you must restrict access to certain areas of the house, stairs, doorways, and so on for baby's own protection. If you want to keep baby confined to one specific area that you know is completely safe but still allow your child to have the freedom to wander, safety gates are key. They are also helpful in keeping your pets separate from your kids. You have the option of installing a temporary or permanent gate. It all depends on what works for your budget and your home. Today, you can buy safety gates that are aesthetically pleasing to the eye as well as eco-friendly. Some look as if they are custom-made for your home.

We had a custom gate made that matched our stairway railing. We installed one at the top and one at the bottom of the stairs. It was helpful because the gate also kept our dog from storming the kids' bedrooms. Now that our kids have grown, of course, we no longer have use for the gates and have had them removed. I bet you can guess where our dog sleeps now. I should've kept those damn gates on!

When it comes to choosing furniture in your home, you may want to think ahead and choose fabrics that are stain-resistant. I learned the hard way that it sucks to clean up baby puke on custom upholstered couches that are not baby-friendly. And the price to have them cleaned sucks even more.

Keeping small toys and objects out of reach is definitely a

smart idea. I was always amazed at how talented our kids were at fitting unexpected things into their mouths. If you are unsure as to what qualifies as a choking hazard, you can easily perform a test with a toilet paper roll. Simply drop any questionable item into a toilet paper tube, and if it passes easily through, then you can be guaranteed that it can get stuck in your kid's throat. It's as simple and scary as that. So be sure to do a sweep of the land a few times a day. Those little critters get their hands on everything in site.

THE WONDERFUL WORLD OF PETS

Introducing them to the kid, yet not neglecting the critters . . .

If pets are an important part of your life, then there is no reason why they can't continue to be so once your baby arrives. You just need to educate yourself on how to handle this new dynamic. It may take some extra work on your part, but at the end of the day the work is well worth it.

If you don't already have a pet, wait until your child is a toddler before you bring a new animal into the home. Three months after Kai was born we decided to get a puppy named Jesse. The perfect addition to our new family, right? Wrong! I can't imagine not having Jesse as part of our family, but between the chewing, the pooing, and the boohooing—and I'm not talking just about Kai—it turned out to be way more work than I'd bargained for. For our next child, I planned ahead. When we had Juliette, I brought home one of her blankets from the hospital so Jesse could get used to her scent.

A baby brings many changes to a household, so try to prep any existing pet for the new arrival. Cats and dogs are sensitive to routines, so by making changes ahead of time, you minimize the chances of your pet resenting your infant when baby is brought home. Here are some tips to get you started:

- Make sure your pet has had contact with other kids, so your child ain't the first who is yanking his or her tail.

- Consider whether your pet's walking, exercise, or feeding schedules need to change to accommodate your baby schedule, and adjust them beforehand.

- You will have less time for your pet after baby's born, so decrease the number of hours you spend with Fido or Whiskers in the weeks before the baby's due so your pet doesn't notice.

- Do not let your pet climb onto baby's furniture or blankets. You do not want your pet getting used to baby's things as play toys.

- Go score a sealed container for soiled diapers. Cats and dogs are very attracted to strong odors (and it gets no stronger than baby poop!) and will drag diapers around the house. You may have enough poop on the walls from baby, so let's not let the family pet contribute.

Your pet is a part of your family, so including him or her is important so your pet doesn't feel neglected or even resent your new addition. Try to have your pet be part of the bonding experience with baby. If you find that you are constantly scolding your pet every time your baby is around, that can make your pet stressed out and perhaps end up not liking your baby.

PLEASE DON'T LET THE DOG
(OR CAT) EAT YOUR BABY

For many of us, our pets are our children. Even after we have human children of our own, the animals we love are still very much a part of the family. However, we do have to make some adjustments once baby crawls into the picture. If you are a dog or cat lover, put into practice the following tips to make sure all your loved ones (human and animal) are existing happily together.

Dogs

- Familiarize your dog with your baby's scent ahead of time. Using a blanket to allow the dog to smell (but not touch) can help establish boundaries and respect for the child. In fact, as you set up the crib and stock up on stuff like baby powder, lotion, and diapers, let your pet come see and smell these things so he or she will get used to their presence.

- No matter how friendly your dog may be, never trust that your pet can be your babysitter. Do not leave the two of them alone at any time. This may sound like a no-brainer, but you'd be surprised how many people just don't get it.

- For the initial introduction it's good to have your dog on a leash just in case your pet gets too eager. Dogs love to be included in everything, especially if you have a Golden like we do, but sometimes their excitement can get out of hand, and it's easy for them to injure your baby just by walking on top of baby or knocking him or her over.

continued . . .

- If you find your dog is barking around the baby, be firm and correct your pet right away. You also want to let your pet know he or she is not allowed to be around the baby without your permission. Teaching this early on is smart and will make you feel more at ease too.

- Evaluate your dog's obedience training. If your pet doesn't respond to basic commands or exhibits any aggressive behavior, seek professional help.

Cats

- Expecting moms should stay away from cat litter as cats can contract toxoplasmosis, a parasite found in the feces. Toxoplasmosis is potentially dangerous to your child if Mom catches it while pregnant, so take some precautions such as having someone else change the litter box daily (that's a plus for Mom, right?) and keeping your cat indoors so it won't hunt any prey that can be infected with the disease.

- Once baby is in the house, trim your cat's claws regularly.

- Put a used receiving blanket or piece of baby's clothes in a quiet area where the cat can investigate it. You want your cat to get used to the smell of your child.

- The myth that cats suck the air out of babies' lungs is indeed an old wives' tale. However, a heat-seeking feline who wants cuddle time could place him- or herself too close to baby's face and make it hard for baby to breathe. A newborn does not have the ability to turn over or even move his or her head at first, so keep kitty out of the crib.

If needed, get extra help from pet-friendly friends, capable neighborhood kids, or dog walking services. At the end of the day you need to figure out a balance to make your pet and your baby both feel like part of the family.

DEAR, SWEET FRIENDS

How to welcome friends into the process and then clear them the hell out!

You don't have to lose yourself when you become a dad, but you may lose a few friends along the way. Some relationships will stand the test of time and others will fall by the wayside.

It may be worth mentioning to your closest buddies that things are gonna change, that you may go from always-f'n-ready-to-rock to missing-in-action for a while. If they are not receptive to the idea that you are settling in (note I didn't say settling *down*) and aren't supportive of you as a dad, then you'll know that putting more energy into the relationship with them will be wasted time. Hopefully they will support your transition into being a father, and if they're really smart, they'll stick around for future advice for their time as dads.

Keep in mind that the friends who seem to have disappeared when your child was born might actually pop back up in the picture later, sometimes in a more significant way than before. Friends who blew you off when you couldn't go out all the time after baby might have a kid of their own a few years later and stumble back into your lives. We had this experience with close friends of ours who are now the godparents to our children (as we are to theirs). That is one of the great things

POST-PREGNANCY SUPPORT GROUPS

As we discussed, many women face severe depression after giving birth. Others simply get into a funk they can't get out of. You may be able to handle this yourself, but don't feel like a failure if you cannot. There are many postpartum depression support groups that are well worth attending, even if you just want to hear others vent so you can assure her she's not so bad off. Talk with your doctor and check the web: postpartum .net and jennyslight.org are good places to start.

about parenting. You never know where you'll end up and with whom.

If you do lose friends, don't be discouraged. Once your little one arrives, you'll be amazed at how easy it is to make new friends, whether you are waiting for your car at the car wash or hanging out at the park. We men can feel a little helpless during the early days of parenting. It's a feeling we're not used to, and it's not always easy to discuss it at home, where we're trying so hard to keep it together. So, man oh man, is it a relief when you run into some random new dad at the soccer field with that now all-too-familiar look of baffled, punched-in-the-gut confusion across his face. You will experience an unspoken bond, one communicated through a knowing nod followed by a "crazy, huh?" or "so what do you do when the poop doesn't stop?" You're together now—that guy could be your next best friend.

TRAVELIN' MAN

Work vs. being there for her. What to do when duty calls . . .

Many dads have to travel as part of their jobs. Early on in the pregnancy, it's not a big deal if you're out of town, as she isn't too dependent on you. By the time she hits the third trimester, she is heavy and hurtin' and can use whatever help you can give. And by the time you two are home with baby, she definitely needs all the help she can get. What do you do if you have to leave town when she needs you the most? You have to earn a living, but you don't wanna leave her side.

There are many ways that you can help out when you have to travel for work after the baby is born. I figured if I couldn't be there in person, I could at least be there in spirit by doing things to help her with the baby while I was gone. It's also not a bad idea to think of some cute little things to keep her feeling loved while you are away. Allow me to share some cool ideas I learned along the way that helped me and my wife cope with the distance:

- Take the lead in finding help for her while you are out of town—family, friends, sitters, trusted neighbors, and so on. This is especially key if you have more than one child. Normal everyday stuff can be overwhelming when she's a new mom, so she will appreciate any support, and you will look like a rock star for having thought of it in advance.

- Skype, email, Facebook, Tweeting, texting, and sexting are all your friends. Schedule times when you can talk via whatever media you prefer and get some face-to-face time if you can. If you already have kids, let them be part of it. If not, use the time for the two of you to enjoy yourselves and have some fun if you catch my drift.

- Thank God for the Internet. These days you can order groceries online, so help out by scheduling an order that can be delivered to the doorstep. Of course, you need to include her in this plan so she knows when it will arrive, but she will appreciate the forethought.

- Leave strategic Post-it notes for your wife to find. This was a favorite of mine. I would take a stack of Post-its and write little notes on them and leave them in areas I knew my wife would find them: in the medicine cabinet, on the refrigerator, in her car, in her wallet, etc. Leave them in places she would and would not expect to find them. Post-its = mucho points.

- Send her flowers and a note to let her know how much she means to you. She will think of you every time she passes by them. And balloons are never a bad idea either. Goofy but effective.

These are just some tips to get you inspired. Traveling can get lonely, but for many families there is no alternative. While it is imperative that you be a good partner to your mate and give Mom a hand, if you are employed then you have a job to do in order to provide for your family. So go do it. Just be sure to make provisions for when you are gone so you are not leaving your partner helpless. Make sure to let her know she is number one while you are away and you are thinking of her. It will pay off when you get back.

SEX AFTER BIRTH
(HMM, THAT SOUNDS AWKWARD . . .)

Yes, there is a sex life for you two after childbirth . . . just
be patient . . ,

So your baby has been born, you made it home, and now you are figuring out your routine . . . which can pretty much be boiled down to sleeping, eating, diaper changing, repeat. To say this new adjustment is chaotic would be an understatement. Did you ever see the Bill Murray flick *Groundhog Day*? For a while that's going to be you. You wake up and repeat the same day over and over and *over* again.

Yet all of this doesn't stop you from wondering when you can start having sex again. And why not? After all, sex is what got you here in the first place, right? Not to mention, it's one of the best ways of connecting with your partner. But be forewarned: at first she may not be up for it, and you too may be so exhausted with your new schedule and focused on your new routine that sex sounds exhausting. Combine this with the fact that your partner may be uncomfortable with the post-birth trauma happening "downtown," especially if she had an episiotomy. The last thing you want to do is contribute to her discomfort, right?

The first few weeks are so exhausting for both of you that mustering up the energy to have sex in the first place will be pretty challenging. But have no fear, this is just a phase. You both will get used to life with baby and your primal urges will soon return . . . often with a vengeance!

Most doctors recommend waiting four to six weeks after giving birth before having sex, especially if your partner had

an episiotomy or a C-section. This time frame allows your partner to heal from the trauma of even a conventional birthing
process, allowing the cervix to close and prevent a uterine
infection. Some women even need stitches due to vaginal tearing during childbirth. The healing of said stitches can result
in scarring or knot-like bumps in that area, so don't wig out.
This is totally normal. If the scars don't fade and she's uncomfortable with them, consider asking her doctor about a steroid
injection to speed along the process.

Keep your antennas up and look for signals. Vaginal sore-
ness and plain ol' exhaustion are likely to be taxing on her, so
you really need to gauge your partner's interest/sex drive as
well. This can be a tough one to wrap your head around, especially if you're thinking from between your legs. Try putting yourself in her shoes in order to understand why sex
might be the last thing on her mind at the moment. You also
want to be sensitive if your partner is experiencing postpartum
depression.

Instead of pressuring her for sex, you can encourage her
to slowly get in the mood. Take the time to cuddle together,
give her a massage, and gently work from there. In fact, easing
back into your sex life can be an opportunity to establish some
new rituals and try fun new stuff. Use this phase to try some
new positions, play some games, explore some fantasies. You've
had a little break from making love, so why not come into it
with a fresh attitude and open mind?

Will it feel different for her, you wonder? Well, after delivery,
decreased muscle tone in the vagina might reduce her pleasure
from friction during sex, which can negatively influence
arousal. But don't worry, this is usually temporary.

DO I HAVE TO WEAR A RUBBER?

Yes. Unless you're hoping to get her pregnant again right away, sex after pregnancy still requires birth control (even if she's breast-feeding). At first, rubbers or spermicides are recommended. Birth control pills or vaginal rings are not recommended early on as they contain estrogen and progestin and can increase risk of blood clots shortly after delivery. For most women, it's all right to begin using birth control pills and other types of combined hormonal birth control six weeks after childbirth.

Once again, we are fortunate as men not to have to endure the physical and emotional discomfort of pregnancy. One of the worst things you can do is to get upset with your partner now for not being in the mood. Think back to the moment your child was emerging from the birth canal and entering your world. Now remember the pained look on your partner's face and the vocal tones that were emerging from her mouth. That should put things in perspective and give you a reason to give her more time if she is not ready. So chill out and put your hand to work. Or better yet, if you are nice to her, maybe she will be willing to use her hand on ya. At least you'll be able to get satisfied, one way or another.

MAN VS. MYTH

Despite what you may have heard,
men can be terrific caregivers too.

There's long been a prevailing belief that men do not know how to care for young children. Bullshit. That may have been true a few generations ago, but we now know that a father can be just as good a primary caregiver as a woman.

Parenting is learned on the job by everyone, moms and dads. Spend time with your kid, and you will become sensitive to what he or she needs. Do what comes natural and go with your gut. There is no one correct definition of what a father is. You have the ability to define fatherhood on your own terms, to craft your own version of a dad to meet the needs of your family. Throughout fatherhood, we men change and grow, we evolve into better people.

Don't let anyone tell you different: your baby needs you too. Just because mom is the one breast-feeding and has that physical connection, do not underestimate your role here. You're an important person in your child's life, and being with you is comforting. Rock baby to sleep, play with baby, and grab that baby bottle when Mom's breasts are sore. In other words, bond with your baby.

"But my dad never did that stuff with me," you say. Maybe that's true, but the role of a father has changed over the years. No longer is it up to the woman to raise the kids while the man brings home the bacon. In fact, I know many modern men who are stay-at-home dads while the wife works a day job. All the more power to both of 'em, I say.

Times have changed, and despite what you may have heard, we men are not destined to be just like our fathers. You love your old man, but your own father doesn't have to be your number one role model for parenting. Any man can be a good father figure, or at least demonstrate admirable attributes. So take the best aspects of the men in your life and combine them into what you want to be for your child, into *who* you want to be for your child.

And remember: while you go through some significant changes as both a couple and individuals, staying true to yourself is part of that journey. You are going to be a dad, but you are still the same dude you were before you started down the road. When fear sets in, simply repeat to yourself, "You don't have to lose who you are when you become a dad." This idea will ground you and keep you on the path of experiencing parenting to the fullest.

Remember . . .

- Hormone changes can find some women facing postpartum depression after giving birth.

- Time to baby-proof your house.

- Just because there's a new baby in the house, don't neglect your pet.

- Allow your friendships to evolve, and be open to making new ones based on parenting experiences.

- If you have to travel for work, make sure you find ways to still participate in the family and make sure Mom knows you are thinking of her.

- Your role as Dad is just as important as Mom's.

- While you need to build a strong partnership with Mom, you don't have to lose your identity when you become a dad.

CHAPTER

6

Happy and Healthy Parenting

I've said it before, but it bears repeating: despite what your sleep-deprived, bleary-eyed friends may ramble at you over beer and nachos, you don't have to lose your identity when you become a dad. Sure, you will have to make some adjustments, and you'll definitely need to make some sacrifices, but that doesn't mean your life ends and fun becomes a faded memory. After the first few months of getting used to your new role and responsibilities, life will settle down to a comfortable tempo and you will get your mojo back. Babysitters equal nights out for you and your lady, and you'll find pushing dinner back to after you put your little one down gives you two plenty of time to be romantic and bond without having to feed mashed food and cheese slices to a crying, soft-skulled munchkin.

Before you know it, your confidence will grow and you will

be out in your hood with your little one in tow on your own, and much less dependent on your lady to solve every problem. As you pass fellow dads strolling along with their kids strapped to their chests or bundled up in the latest Bugaboo stroller, you will exchange a knowing, approving nod as you pass each other by, letting each other know that you are both a part of the tribe. You, my friend, are special. And now you are a dad. Cheers!

Don't worry if there are bumps in the road. The first day I mustered up the courage to take my son out for a walk with a friend was a bit nerve-wracking, to say the least. I put Kai in a baby carrier and off we went. Not even halfway down the block Kai started crying uncontrollably. My friend who was not yet a dad was with me and he had no idea what was going on. In fact, the crying really seemed to stress him out. I tried my best to act cool amid the pouring sweat that was streaming down my face. I tried bouncing, singing, distracting Kai any way I could. Eventually I discovered that the reason he was crying was because I had accidentally put both of his legs into the same pant leg of his jeans. Wow, did I feel like a dumbass! But once I figured it out, he stopped his crying and I trudged on. Figuring that out for myself made me feel confident that I could handle him on my own. If I had panicked and gone back home to Meredith with my tail between my legs, I would've felt like such a loser. I laugh about it today, but in that moment figuring it out for myself made a difference. I'm not suggesting you parent without the help of others, of course, but you are more competent than you think.

In fact, the usefulness of what you've learned during your wife's pregnancy doesn't have to stop when the baby's born. The very principles and behavior that made you a good partner during your wife's pregnancy will also serve you well as your child grows older. Patience, communicating, helping around the house, staying educated on what is going on with your loved ones, and being emotionally and physically available are all attributes that will benefit you as both a father and a husband in the many happy years to come. Quite the payoff, huh?

So here are some ways you can apply what you learned over the past nine months to continue being a good partner. These are issues we have covered from the perspective of an expecting father, but now they can be reapplied and used as guidelines for what comes next.

GET IT OUT

The key to a strong relationship is good communication. Keeping these lines open is vital. Especially once the newborn arrives. Now, that doesn't mean just say whatever is on your mind with no filter whatsoever. But bottling up our emotions only leads to outbursts, resentment, and acting out. Voicing feelings right off the bat will eliminate that awkward tension. Using examples of why you feel the way you do, and not just lashing out with emotion, is also helpful. Trying to help your partner understand why you are hurt or upset, and discussing how you could avoid going down this path again are helpful ways to avoid repeat behavior.

Same thing when you're being a dad. You can't just yell at your kid as soon as he or she does wrong. You have to talk to your child and set guidelines and restrictions so your child understands boundaries. Communicate with your child.

Talking about issues the first time they occur generally leads to much less frustration if they happen again. And if you don't have a bunch of anger bottled up inside you from not saying anything the first time, you are less likely to explode the next time.

LISTEN, STOP FIXING

As men we are programmed to be problem solvers. We want to be heroes. Unfortunately this behavior drives my wife nuts! She doesn't want me to figure out her problem or magically take away her feelings, she just wants me to listen. It's hard at first, but once you get the hang of it, it makes things run much more smoothly.

When we become fathers, this urge to problem solve gets even stronger. We are literally heroes to our children. Real-life supermen. It's hard not to want always to say and do the right thing to make the tears go away. But sometimes kids just need to vent too. Even children need to get their frustrations and emotions out. If we can easily solve their problems, great. Letting them get it out, work it out, and solve their own problems can work wonders too.

USE THE PAUSE BUTTON

This is a no-brainer, but don't be fooled. It's probably the most difficult of all the tips on this list. We often find ourselves wanting to prove a point and have our voices heard at all costs.

Instead, take a moment to think things through. It'll make you respond more responsibly and less defensively. There is no way you are going to succeed if you don't understand where your partner is coming from and take these factors into consideration. Take a moment, breathe, think, process, and then respond. You will be glad you did.

This is a lesson you can apply to being a father and to life in general. Taking a moment to collect your thoughts, to collect yourself, is never a bad idea. Too often we leap to conclusions or act purely out of emotion in a situation. A self-imposed time-out can add some fresh perspective and allow some of the anger or frustration to slip away. At that point you are acting on reason. Arm reason with facts and you have all the ammo you need for any conflict.

KEEP THINGS FRESH

Keep things fresh, and don't take your relationship for granted. This is a lesson we dudes could learn long before becoming a dad. Get in the habit of surprising your partner, whether it is with spontaneous weekend getaways, cooking her favorite dinners, coming home with flowers or balloons, or whatever small tokens you can think of to let her know how much she means to you. Never underestimate the power of a small, sweet gesture. Practice early, so once the baby arrives it'll be second nature.

And once baby grows up, having a father that is always

coming up with cool, fun ideas is quite awesome. Being that dad that takes the team out for pizza after the games, spontaneously hits an amusement park or movie once in a while, or instigates neat arts and crafts activities together is a great thing. Make your kid pancakes one morning. Take some fruit and make smoothies in the blender. Offer to take your kid and his or her friend on a hike. Be that guy who makes his kid's life an adventure.

TACKLE FEAR

Sometimes we freak out about the idea of being a dad. Can I do this? Can I afford this? Will I be good at it? These are normal fears, not reality.

It's hard to jump right in when the baby is born, since we don't get to physically connect like our pregnant partner. But finding ways to try to connect is helpful. Get involved in your partner's process as much as possible. Be curious, ask questions about her experience, and attend as many doctor visits and classes with her as you can. This will ease you into your new role and slowly begin to eliminate your fear. Remember what *Schoolhouse Rock* taught us: knowledge is power.

As your child grows, a whole new set of fears will kick in. Who are these new friends? Who is my kid hanging out with at school? At what age is a sleepover okay? When do we allow our teenager to date? Are there older teens at those parties our kid goes to? These are fears every parent faces. The best thing you can do is start dealing with them early on. Talk to your partner about them and come up with solutions together. You are a team now more than ever and have to make the right choices for your child. You won't make the best decisions if you are acting out of fear. Break down what scares you and confront it head on. Remember, it's all the same stuff our parents had to deal with when we were kids (school, responsibility, money, bad crowds, sex, drugs, and so on), and we turned out all right.

PRACTICE ROMANCE 101

Oftentimes being a parent can put a damper on the romance in a relationship. But, as guys, we can make an effort to keep it alive. Don't take your relationship for granted just because you have a kid. Sex can be an incredible way to bond with your partner and remind her that she is still a woman, not just a mom. Make sure she feels sexy and attractive. It also happens to be one of the most fun ways to work on your relationship!

But sex is not the only way to keep your romance alive. Think back to those early years of courtship and bring that feeling back. As we just discussed, surprises, dates, thoughtful gifts, little notes, random calls or texts with messages of love— I can't emphasize enough how important these things are. Make her feel special. Go the extra mile. It will make you feel good about yourself too. Few things are as fulfilling as knowing you are the best man for your woman.

ASK QUESTIONS

A key factor in being a helpful parent is to seek advice from other parents. Accept that you don't know everything and don't be afraid to seek counsel from others. More often than not, experience is the only way to learn, so it is helpful to talk to some experienced parents ahead of time to prepare yourself. Don't wait until you are in the thick of it. Ask questions *before* you are inadvertently stepping into quicksand. Get ahead of the game and seek out advice. You have a whole army of people in your life who have gone through this and are generally happy to dole out advice. From your friends and coworkers, to your parents and family, to the butcher behind the counter at Ralphs or the secretary with flowery-framed pictures of her kids on her desk, there are plenty of parents out there who can help you out and will be happy to do so. Don't be afraid to use your resources. Put your ego aside.

You are in uncharted waters, my friend, and you just don't have all the answers. But that's okay, it's a big club and you are about to become a member. This is good advice not only when she is expecting, but after the baby is born and you are in full swing as a parent. We men assume we know it all. We don't. And that's okay. We can learn.

TEMPER YOUR EXPECTATIONS

I got into trouble many times because I expected Meredith to handle things after she got pregnant the way she would have before she was carrying. Once your partner is pregnant, don't assume she is going to react to things the way she used to. She is going through all sorts of physical and emotional changes, so bear with her and cut her some slack. Always act as if you are doing things for the first time and run it by her first. Believe me, it'll save you the hours of "disagreeing" later on.

Tempering the expectations you put on your child is not a bad idea as well. Too often fathers have a preconceived notion as to how their kid will turn out. "I want my boy to be a star!" "Tommy will be the best damn soccer player there is." It's good to set goals for your child, and definitely good to get your child involved in activities and teams, but don't take it too seriously, Dad. Let kids be kids. Let them screw up sometimes. Let them be who they want to be. Give them the opportunity, and children will often surpass even our wildest expectations.

IT'S ALL ABOUT WE, NOT ME

Just as pregnancy takes teamwork, so does parenting. It's not all about you anymore, pal. Start early on making choices that are in the best interests of you both, so that it will have become second nature once the baby arrives. For instance, maybe it's not so smart to commit to those Lakers tickets when your partner is vomiting incessantly. Seems like a no-brainer, right? Believe me, not all guys will think that one through.

Remembering the days when it was the two of you against the world is also helpful when it comes to being a team player. As the reality of becoming a parent settles in, it's good to remember that this woman is still your best friend and life mate, and the sexiest female to allow you to have sex with her on a regular basis. In fact, once you're a parent, your relationship can soar to new heights and you two will share happiness you could never have imagined before you knocked her up. So don't forget that you are a team for a reason: because you two are meant for each other and complement each other in incredible ways. That won't change. In fact, it'll get better.

COMPROMISE

This one goes without saying. You will be making many compromises when you become a dad. It's part of the job. Depending on how your partner handles her pregnancy, these compromises may begin early on or may not affect you until the baby arrives. Once your newborn arrives, choosing what's best for all three of you will become second nature and it will make you a more responsible dad. It is a mistake to think that having to bend on issues is a sign of weakness on your part. You and your partner are a team now more than ever, and both of you need to put what is best for the child over your own interest. Sometimes what's best for the child is simply for you to shut up, give in, and do what needs to get done. If it means you don't get to eat what you want when you want, or can't go see that new Jason Statham movie you want to ('cause you know he's gonna beat the stuffing out of a whole bunch of bad dudes and it's gonna rock), that's okay. There will be plenty of opportunities to do that stuff later on.

Compromise does not mean giving up something forever. It's more like a give-and-take. I've certainly made compromises, but oddly enough, something better and more amazing than I ever imagined was often the result. Be open to it. You never know where you will end up. Staying positive will help to make the road easier and more enjoyable.

This goes back to my original philosophy: you don't have to lose who you are when you become a dad. You'll often find that what you originally perceive as a compromise or sacrifice is actually merely a choice you are making for the betterment of your family. It's cool, dude. That's what we parents do. That's what makes us so awesome. Without even being aware of it we have grown into slightly less selfish people. Amazing, eh?

Conclusion
Welcome to the Club

Despite all the information I've shared in this book, and despite the nine whole months you have to get ready, no one can truly explain the feeling of becoming a dad until you actually experience it yourself. You arm yourself with all this information, and then when that moment happens, everything flies out the window and nothing else matters except this small baby in front of you. All that stress about being a dad was based on fear and the unknown. Now you are here in the moment and there is just . . . this child . . . this glow.

Dude, it will change you forever.

Life is about experiencing things, and you've just experienced one of the biggest things life has to offer. There's nothing like living through that actual moment. Everything is put into perspective. And *that* is "The Club."

Parents talk about "The Club" like it's a do-gooder secret society or some understood, underlying warmth we parents share like a really wimpy version of The Force or something. No. The Club for us dads means we all went through that same awakening, that same moment where everything clicked and we saw the proverbial light. It's that nod you give every dad you ever see for the rest of your life that's holding his kid's hand or carrying a diaper bag. "That's cool. He's doing it." *That* is The Club.

You're part of this movement that's happening, this generation of dads who are saying, "We can handle it." It is a really powerful thing; kind of the men's version of the Women's Movement. You're re-creating a role. It's about family, a team, not just one person doing everything while the other watches *Seinfeld* reruns.

You are a father now.

You are evolving as a man.

It's a beautiful thing, dude.

Dude Weekly Pregnancy Updates Calendar

Week 1 & 2—This is the time where your mate has been ovulating, so now would be the time to do the deed (or was the time you already did the deed). Remember to keep your jewels cool. No hot baths! Since pregnancy is determined by the date of your partner's last menstrual cycle, these two weeks are included in that timeline. Nothing much to report here but hopefully your partner will begin to take her folic acid to keep the baby developing properly.

Week 3—Sperm and egg have met and now you are gonna be a dad. Way to go! This is the time she'll take a pregnancy test. Right now your little one is just a blob about the size of a pin. Crazy to think how fast it grows in just over forty weeks.

Week 4—Not much physically has happened to your partner yet, but internally the implantation process has begun. That fertilized egg is burrowing itself into the lining of your partner's uterus. By the end of the first month the amniotic sac forms around the egg to protect it as it grows. The placenta also develops. A primitive face starts to take shape with large dark circles for eyes. Your baby's mouth, throat, and lower jaw are developing. Blood cells begin to form and circulation will begin. Your little one is about a quarter inch long, almost the size of an orange seed or a grain of rice.

Week 5—This is the time where you may be able to hear your baby's heartbeat, so make sure you join her for her next doctor appointment. Your partner may begin to feel symptoms such as nausea, exhaustion, hormonal imbalance, and mood swings. From here on out, dude, you need to be extra sensitive. Oh, one more thing—she's probably gonna start peeing a lot.

Week 6—You may notice your partner more sensitive to smells. Morning sickness most likely will have kicked in, and if your partner is able to hold it down, she may notice some signs of weight gain and fuller breasts. Remember, they're not for you to play with! Right now until about fourteen weeks your little one is susceptible to anything that can affect normal growth, so this is the vulnerable period when many choose to wait to tell others they are pregnant. So both of you need to decide if you want to tell anyone at all or just those closest to you.

Week 7—Eating bland may be the only way to survive at this point. Make sure your partner is drinking enough fluids too. The bathroom may be her new refuge until these pregnancy symptoms subside. Be understanding at this time. Eliminate smells that bug her (cologne, aftershave, etc.) and suggest protein smoothies as a source of energy and relief from nausea.

Week 8—Right now fingers and toes are beginning to form on your little one. Your little pea is finally starting to take shape and look more baby-like as the nose, lips, and eyelids begin to take shape. Your partner is still battling morning sickness, so continue to be there for her and avoid pissing her off.

Week 9—Dude, the baby's toes are starting to form. Woo-hoo! Patience is going to be your best friend right now as your partner is still battling the nausea beast. Don't be offended if she yacks on you mid-conversation. A lot of stuff is happening inside her. By the way, she may also be farting a lot.

Week 10—While numerous changes are occurring to your baby—like its head becoming rounder and the neck beginning to develop—your partner is not going to feel much different. Try to up the effort to soothe your nauseous lady. Encourage her to eat small meals instead of big ones. Offer her a foot rub to distract the dizziness and fatigue. Stock up on peppermint tea and ginger. She will love you for it.

Week 11—It's official: you can now call your growing baby a fetus. Sounds weird, doesn't it? Important things are developing like the penis and testicles if it's a boy or the clitoris if it's a girl. Not to mention that he or she measures about two inches in size. It's possible the nausea is starting to wind down for your lady. Thank God! But don't get too excited; it will rear its head once more come the third trimester. Keep working to make your partner comfortable and relaxed. She should be getting her energy back pretty soon.

Week 12—Your baby is about the size of a plum now, which means your partner will most likely be showing at this point. If you have not yet spilled the beans, you better think fast if someone puts you on the spot. Your baby now has a human profile and fingernails. Cool, right?

Week 13—This week your little one's fingerprints are actually being formed. Not to mention that the veins and organs are visible through your baby's thin skin. This week is also the last of your partner's first trimester. The chance of a miscarriage reduces greatly from this point on. The tide should be turning and taking her nausea along with it, but keep an eye out for dizzy spells, as your partner may still be feeling weak.

Week 14—Get this, your little one can pee now and most likely is able to suck his or her own thumb. Cool, right? Your partner's energy should be returning soon. It may be smart to suggest a workout routine together. Foot rubs are a good idea this week, and if she is able to tolerate smells now, perhaps a homecooked meal is the way to go. Cooked by *you*, that is.

Week 15—Baby is about the size of an orange now and weighs about one-and-three-quarter ounces. Your partner has been gaining weight (around five pounds or so), so be sensitive to comments about her looks. Whatever you do, do not say she is fat! But you already know that by now, right? Compliment her on her looks to keep her feeling positive and sexy.

Week 16—Most likely your partner is experiencing that "pregnancy glow" right about now. Finally, right? Your baby is starting to hear sounds too, so warm up that singing voice and start talking to your lady's belly. Don't judge yourself. At first it seems weird, but as time goes on and your baby grows, your bond will too. Trust me, we've all done it.

Week 17—Your little dude's cartilage is turning into bones and he's putting on fat. This is all good. Meanwhile, your partner may be feeling some sciatic nerve pain in her legs and noticing stretch marks. Be sensitive and give her a rub with coconut oil to give her some relief. Now is a good time to start thinking about childbirth classes.

Week 18—The second trimester ultrasound can be scheduled now. Be sure you are available to be there. Your partner's back may be aching now too, so be sure to pitch in with chores around the house and give her a back rub, dammit!

Week 19—Your baby is now covered in a cheesy white substance called Vernix caseosa. This stuff protects baby from the amniotic fluid surrounding him or her. Leg cramps may be setting in for your partner, so be sure to help her get some relief (hint, hint: perhaps a massage?). Keep her comfortable, especially since her belly is beginning to grow.

Week 20—This gooey black stuff called meconium is brewing inside your little one. It's totally normal. On another, brighter note, your partner is halfway there. She's probably gained at least ten pounds by now. From this point on to keep her strength up she may require more iron than she's been getting. Nurture your inner chef, dude, and cook away. She'll love you for it.

Week 21—This week your baby is about the size of a pomegranate, about ten and a half inches. You may be able to feel the baby kicking inside your partner's belly. Grab a children's book like *Goodnight Moon* and start reading to her belly as you unwind in bed. Get into a bonding-with-baby bedtime routine early on.

Week 22—One pregnancy symptom your lady may be experiencing this week is an increased libido. Woo-hoo! Go for it, dude! And don't worry, you will not hit the baby with your tool. If only you were *that* big, right?

Week 23—You may notice your partner being a bit more forgetful than normal. No worries. It's just another symptom of her pregnancy, so cut her some slack. If only we men could use that as our excuse, right?

Week 24—It's around this time that she'll need to undergo a glucose screening test, basically a blood exam that tests for gestational diabetes, a high-blood-sugar condition related to pregnancy. It's times like these, while she waits for the results, that offering a shoulder to lean on is important.

Week 25—Dude, press your ear to your partner's belly. You hear it? That's your baby's heartbeat. Crazy, right? Remember to encourage your partner to drink lots of water to stay hydrated. You can leave some extra water bottles around the house just to remind her.

Week 26—As time goes on and your partner's belly continues to grow, she is definitely going to feel exhausted and achy. It would be nice to surprise her with a warm bath to soothe her aching muscles and some relaxing music to enjoy.

Week 27—This week marks the close of the second trimester. Time is flyin' (at least for you, that is). Your baby weighs about two pounds at this point. Pretty cool. If you are feeling anxiety about your new role as dad, now is a good time to start chatting with fellow dads or your close buds. Having an outlet is important.

Week 28—Congrats! This week is the start of the third trimester. You are almost there. If you haven't already signed up for childbirth classes, there's no reason to wait any longer. Consider infant CPR as part of the education. Preparation is the key to parenting.

Week 29—Now is not a bad time to start discussing who will join you in the delivery room. Remember to be open to letting her close friends be a part of the delivery. Believe me, you will want the extra support.

Week 30—Heads up, dude. Those mood swings may be back. Do not even attempt to fight back if you find yourself in the doghouse. No man has been known to defeat the hormone beast.

Week 31—As your baby's growth continues (he or she is now about the size of a coconut), there will be a lot of movement happening inside. In fact, those Braxton Hicks contractions I mentioned may be showing up, not to mention your partner feeling out of breath. Keep communication open and be a support to her symptoms by taking over if need be (for example, calling the doctor if she's feeling more pain in her uterus than normal). She is really gonna need you in the coming weeks, more than ever.

Week 32—Dude, three pounds. That's how much your little one weighs at this point, give or take a few ounces. A neat fact: at this stage your baby experiences rapid eye movement, which signifies he or she may be dreaming when sleeping. Cool, huh? Keep an eye on your partner this week as she gets to the home stretch. She's probably feeling really tired these days. Remind her to take a load off and chill.

Week 33—Your little one is about seventeen inches long at this point. How the hell does that baby fit inside your partner, right? Well, that explains why she may be more irritable these days. She may also be starting the "nesting" phase in preparation for the birth. Remind her to take it easy. Rest is important from here on out.

Week 34—If it's a boy, this is the week his testes descend, forming his scrotum! Meanwhile, your partner is continuing to feel sluggish. Be patient with her. You are almost there.

Week 35—So did you discuss whether or not your partner will be getting an epidural? Now is a good time, though I'd advise letting her make the final decision. After all, she's the one who will be enduring the pain. If she doesn't want it, then get ready to help her through a wild ride of pain!

Week 36—Dude, did you pack your bag for the hospital yet? If not, what are you waiting for? Get it done now!

Week 37—Congratulations. Your baby is now full term. He or she should arrive any time now. Did you map out the route to the hospital yet? Is your car filled with enough gas to get you there? If not, get to it!

Week 38—Your baby may still be cooking, so most likely you are on edge with excitement waiting for him or her to come out. It's going to get chaotic once it's time to head to the hospital, so you may want to make a list of those you need to contact to share the good news once the baby is born. The last thing you need now is your mom pissed at you for forgetting to call her.

Week 39—You're closing in on the sleepless nights, so rest up while you can (unless of course your little one has already arrived—in that case, congrats!!!!).

Week 40—This is it, dude. If it's not now, well, it could be any day or up to two more weeks from now. Hang in there and practice coaching your lady. Be supportive, as your partner may be frustrated that the due date came and went. You baby is probably seven to eight pounds now. Damn, hope the contractions kick in soon! Good luck.

Sources

CHAPTER 0: BEFORE THE COUNTDOWN BEGINS

MISCELLANEOUS LUPUS FACTS

"Lupus: Definition." Mayo Clinic. Oct. 26, 2011. mayoclinic.org/diseases-conditions/lupus/basics/definition/con-20019676.

"Lupus." *Health*. health.com/health/lupus.

Murkoff, Heidi, and Sharon Mazel. *What to Expect When You're Expecting* (New York: Workman, 2008), 526.

Roizen, Michael F., and Mehmet C. Oz. *YOU: Having a Baby: The Owner's Manual to a Happy and Healthy Pregnancy* (New York: Free Press, 2009), 48, 379.

"What Is Lupus?" Medical News Today. August 2013. medicalnewstoday.com/info/lupus.

MOM, TREAT THAT BODY RIGHT

"Getting Healthy Before Pregnancy." March of Dimes. October 2013. marchofdimes.com/pregnancy/getting-healthy-before -pregnancy.aspx.

Murkoff and Mazel. *What to Expect When You're Expecting*, 2–13.

"Plan and Prepare for Pregnancy." Ohio State University. medical center.osu.edu/patientcare/healthcare_services/womens_ health/prevention/pregnancy/Pages/index.aspx.

Roizen and Oz. *YOU: Having a Baby*, 292, 293, 303, 304, 305.

"Seventeen Things You Should Do Before You Try to Get Pregnant." BabyCenter. babycenter.com/0_seventeen-things-you-should -do-before-you-try-to-get-pregnan_7171.bc.

PREPPING FOR IMPREGNATING

Lucille, Holly. Email interview. January 12, 2014.

Murkoff and Mazel. *What to Expect When You're Expecting*, 2–13.

Norrgard, Karen. "Diagnosing Down Syndrome, Cystic Fibrosis, Tay-Sachs Disease and Other Genetic Disorders." Nature Education. 2008. nature.com/scitable/topicpage/diagnosing-down -syndrome-cystic-fibrosis-tay-sachs-646.

Roizen and Oz. *YOU: Having a Baby*, 292, 293, 303, 304, 305.

DUDE, TREAT YOUR BODY RIGHT

"Health Tip: Pre-Pregnancy Health for Men." *U.S. News & World Report*, April 30, 2008. health.usnews.com/usnews/health/ healthday/080430/health-tip-pre-pregnancy-health-for-men .htm.

"Pre-Conception Health for Men." American Pregnancy Association. November 2012. americanpregnancy.org/gettingpregnant/ menpreconception.htm.

Roizen and Oz. *YOU: Having a Baby*, 383, 386, 387, 388.

KEEP COOL

Fisch, Harry. "When Hot Tubs Aren't Such a Hot Idea." *The Dr. Oz Show*, Feb. 9, 2010. doctoroz.com/blog/harry-fisch-md/when-hot-tubs-aren-t-such-hot-idea.

Kain, Erica. "Trying to Get Pregnant? 10 Proven Sperm Killers." MSN Healthy Living healthyliving.msn.com/health-wellness/trying-to-get-pregnant-10-proven-sperm-killers.

Weschler, Toni. "Should We Steer Clear of the Hot Tub While Trying to Get Pregnant?" BabyCenter. babycenter.com/404_should-we-steer-clear-of-the-hot-tub-while-trying-to-get-pre_1336309.bc.

DID YOU KNOW?

"Fertilization." Mayo Clinic. mayoclinic.org/health/medical/IM01237.

"Low Sperm Count." Mayo Clinic, September 22, 2012. mayoclinic.org/health/low-sperm-count/DS01049.

"Low Sperm Count Causes." Mayo Clinic, September 22, 2012. mayoclinic.org/health/low-sperm-count/DS01049/DSECTION=causes.

"Male Infertility." Planned Parenthood. plannedparenthood.org/health-topics/mens-sexual-health/male-infertility-22754.htm.

Roizen and Oz. *YOU: Having a Baby*, 383, 384, 386.

IT'S A CELEBRATION, Y'ALL! . . . OR IS IT?

Horan, Molly. "23 Creative Ways to Tell the World You're Having a Baby." Buzzfeed.com. November 2, 2012. buzzfeed.com/mollykateri/23-creative-ways-to-tell-the-world-youre-having-a-421u.

SEX: WILL WE EVER HAVE IT AGAIN?

Burns, Ami. "What Happens After Your Mucus Plug Comes Out?" *Parents*. parents.com/advice/pregnancy-birth/giving-birth/what-happens-after-your-mucus-plug-comes-out.

Charlish, Anne, and Kim Davies. *The Complete Book of Natural Pregnancy and Childcare* (Leicester, UK: Lorenz Books, 2008), 14–16, 20, 134.

"Labor Contractions." Sutter Health. babies.sutterhealth.org/laboranddelivery/labor/ld_contractns.html.

"Mucus Plug." eMedTV. July 17, 2013. pregnancy.emedtv.com/mucus-plug/mucous-plug.html.

Murkoff and Mazel. *What to Expect When You're Expecting*, 184, 185, 255, 258, 463, 464.

Roizen and Oz. *YOU: Having a Baby*, 172–175, 184, 185, 196.

"Sex During Pregnancy." BabyCenter. babycenter.com/sex-during-pregnancy.

"Sex During Pregnancy." March of Dimes. March 2009. marchofdimes.com/pregnancy/sex-during-pregnancy.aspx.

"Sex During Pregnancy: What's OK, What's Not." Mayo Clinic, July 24, 2012. mayoclinic.org/sex-during-pregnancy/art-20045318.

"What Is the Amniotic Sac?" National Health Service (UK). December 15, 2013. nhs.uk/chq/Pages/2310.aspx?CategoryID=54.

DID YOU KNOW?

Keenihan, Sarah. "Seminal Fluid, Not Just Sperm, Enables Pregnancy." *Cosmos.* November 28, 2012. cosmosmagazine.com/news/seminal-fluid-not-just-sperm-critical-pregnancy.

"Semen." Encyclopedia Britannica. britannica.com/EBchecked/topic/533862/semen.

THE CYCLE OF THE MENSTRUATION CYCLE

Murkoff and Mazel. *What to Expect When You're Expecting*, 8, 9, 17, 20, 21.

"Normal Menstrual Cycle." WebMD. March 22, 2011. women.webmd.com/tc/normal-menstrual-cycle-topic-overview.

"Menstrual Cycle: What's Normal, What's Not." Mayo Clinic. April 16, 2013. mayoclinic.org/menstrual-cycle/art-20047186.

Roizen and Oz. *YOU: Having a Baby*, 195, 386.

SPOTTING

"Abnormal Vaginal Bleeding." WebMD. June 20, 2011. women
.webmd.com/tc/abnormal-vaginal-bleeding-topic-overview.
Murkoff and Mazel. *What to Expect When You're Expecting*, 237, 343.
"Vaginal Bleeding or Spotting During Pregnancy" BabyCenter.
November 2012. babycenter.com/0_vaginal-bleeding-or
-spotting-during-pregnancy_3081.bc.

CHAPTER 1: THE FIRST TRIMESTER

"The First Trimester: Your Baby's Growth and Development in Early
Pregnancy" WebMD. July 8, 2013. webmd.com/baby/
1to3-months.
"First Trimester Symptoms." Parenting.com. parenting.com/article/
first-trimester-symptoms&lnk=mostpop&loc=fertility.
Murkoff and Mazel. *What to Expect When You're Expecting*, 59, 60, 135.
"Pregnancy Week by Week: First Trimester." Mayo Clinic. March
19, 2011. mayoclinic.org/healthy-living/pregnancy-week-by
-week/basics/healthy-pregnancy/hlv-20049471
Roizen and Oz. *YOU: Having a Baby*, 295, 303, 304.

WHERE ARE WE NOW?

"Morning Sickness: Causes, Concerns, Treatments." BabyCenter.
March 2013. babycenter.com/morning-sickness.
"Pregnancy Week by Week (First, Second, and Third Trimester)."
Medicinet.com. medicinenet.com/pregnancy/article.htm.
"Pregnancy Week by Week: First Trimester." Mayo Clinic. March
19, 2011. mayoclinic.org/healthy-living/pregnancy-week
-by-week/basics/healthy-pregnancy/hlv-20049471.

HORMONES, HORMONES, HORMONES

Charlish and Davies. *The Complete Book of Natural Pregnancy and
Childcare*, 16, 28, 50, 70, 82, 90, 120, 122.

"Guide to Pregnancy Hormones." What to Expect. whattoexpect
.com/pregnancy/pregnancy-health/pregnancy-hormones.aspx.

"Heightened Sense of Smell." PregnancyCorner. pregnancycorner
.com/pregnant/pregnancy-symptoms/heightened-sense-of
-smell.html.

Hochwald, Lambeth. "A Cheat Sheet to Pregnancy Hormones."
Parents. 2011. parents.com/pregnancy/my-life/emotions/
understanding-pregnancy-hormones.

"Mood Swings During Pregnancy." BabyCenter. babycenter.com/
0_mood-swings-during-pregnancy_253.bc.

Roizen and Oz. *YOU: Having a Baby,* 153, 162, 167, 211, 383, 384.

WONDERFUL WORLD OF HORMONES

Szabo, Liz. "Dads' Hormones Change, Too, During Pregnancy."
USA Today. June 14, 2010. usatoday30.usatoday.com/news/
health/2010-06-15-daddybrain15_cv_N.htm.

THE PORCELAIN THRONE (AKA YOUR WIFE'S NEW BEST FRIEND)

"About Hyperemesis Gravidarum." HER Foundation. April 18,
2013. helpher.org/hyperemesis-gravidarum.

Charlish and Davies. *The Complete Book of Natural Pregnancy and
Childcare,* 89, 111, 223, 445.

Eng, Heather. "15 Tips for Dealing with Morning Sickness." *Parents.*
parents.com/pregnancy/my-body/morning-sickness/morning
-sickness.

"Hyperemesis Gravidarum." National Institutes of Health. November 8, 2012. nlm.nih.gov/medlineplus/ency/article/001499.htm.

"Morning Sickness." American Pregnancy Association. american
pregnancy.org/pregnancyhealth/morningsickness
.html.

"Morning Sickness." BabyCenter. March 2013. babycenter.com/
morning-sickness.

"Morning Sickness: Definition." Mayo Clinic, October 4, 2011. mayoclinic.org/health/morning-sickness/DS01150.

Murkoff and Mazel. *What to Expect When You're Expecting*, 130, 131, 139, 545.

Roizen and Oz. *YOU: Having a Baby*, 76, 77, 127, 268.

"10 Remedies for Pregnancy Nausea." SheKnows: Pregnancy and Baby. pregnancyandbaby.com/pregnancy/articles/942687/10-remedies-for-pregnancy-nausea.

WHAT TO DO?

Bingham, Helena. "Eat Small Meals Every Few Hours." What to Eat When Pregnant. whattoeatwhenpregnant.co.uk/eat-small-meals-every-few-hours.

"Losing Weight While Pregnant." What to Eat When Pregnant. whattoeatwhenpregnant.us/losing-weight-while-pregnant.html.

"What Not to Eat When Pregnant." WebMD. March 28, 2013. webmd.com/baby/ss/slideshow-what-not-to-eat-when-pregnant.

"What to Eat During Pregnancy." Medical News Today. July 15, 2013. medicalnewstoday.com/articles/246404.php.

SUPER POWERS 'N' MOOD SWINGS

"Guide to Pregnancy Hormones." What to Expect. whattoexpect.com/pregnancy/pregnancy-health/pregnancy-hormones.aspx.

Hochwald, Lambeth. "A Cheat Sheet to Pregnancy Hormones." *Parents*. 2011. parents.com/pregnancy/my-life/emotions/understanding-pregnancy-hormones.

"Mood Swings." American Pregnancy Association. January 2013. americanpregnancy.org/pregnancyhealth/moodswings.html.

"Mood Swings in Pregnancy." BabyCenter. April 2012. babycentre.co.uk/a253/mood-swings-in-pregnancy.

Murkoff and Mazel. *What to Expect When You're Expecting*, 15, 130, 133.

Robinson, Holly. "Why Is My Pregnant Wife So Moody?" *American Baby*. September 2004. parents.com/pregnancy/my-life/emotions/pregnancy-mood-swings.

Roizen and Oz. *YOU: Having a Baby*, 137, 145–148, 153, 162, 165, 167, 172, 173.

"Your Pregnancy: 10 Things That Might Surprise You About Being Pregnant." KidsHealth. kidshealth.org/parent/pregnancy_center/your_pregnancy/pregnancy.html.

DIZZY MISS LIZZY

"Fetal Development: The Second Trimester." Mayo Clinic. December 4, 2012. mayoclinic.org/fetal-development/art-20046151.

Murkoff and Mazel. *What to Expect When You're Expecting*, 236, 237.

CHAPTER 2: THE SECOND TRIMESTER

"Fetal Development: Second Trimester." American Pregnancy Association. January 2013. americanpregnancy.org/duringpregnancy/fetaldevelopment2.htm.

"Fetal Development: The Second Trimester." Mayo Clinic. December 4, 2012. mayoclinic.org/fetal-development/art-20046151.

Murkoff and Mazel. *What to Expect When You're Expecting*, 66, 244, 245.

Roizen and Oz. *YOU: Having a Baby*, 296, 301, 302, 304, 305.

"Second Trimester of Pregnancy." WebMD. July 20, 2012. webmd.com/baby/guide/second-trimester-of-pregnancy.

"Second Trimester Symptoms." Parenting.com. parenting.com/article/Pregnancy-Symptoms-Second-Trimester.

ULTRASOUND: THE MUST-SEE MOVIE OF THE YEAR!

"All About Ultrasounds." BabyCenter. February 2012. babycenter.com/0_all-about-ultrasounds_329.bc.

Charlish and Davies. *The Complete Book of Natural Pregnancy and Childcare*, 83, 85, 87, 104, 107, 119, 169.

Murkoff and Mazel. *What to Expect When You're Expecting*, 62, 64, 65, 245.

"Ultrasound: Definition." Mayo Clinic. February 23, 2012. mayoclinic.org/health/ultrasound/MY00308.

"Ultrasound in Pregnancy." The Society of Obstetricians and Gynaecologists of Canada. sogc.org/publications/ultrasound-in -pregnancy.

"What Is Gestational Diabetes?" American Diabetes Association. November 26, 2013. diabetes.org/diabetes-basics/gestational/ what-is-gestational-diabetes.html.

SEX STATUS

"Fetal Development: The Second Trimester." Mayo Clinic. December 4, 2012. mayoclinic.org/fetal-development/art-20046151.

Murkoff and Mazel. *What to Expect When You're Expecting*, 62, 66, 245.

Pryor, Elizabeth. "Q&A: How Soon Can You Find Out Baby's Sex?" *American Baby*. parents.com/pregnancy/my-baby/gender -prediction/finding-out-babys-sex.

SOME FOOD ADVICE FOR MOM

Charlish and Davies. *The Complete Book of Natural Pregnancy and Childcare*, 30, 36, 37, 41, 310, 311.

"If You're Pregnant, You Can Eat for Two, Right?" WebMD. July 1, 2010. webmd.com/baby/features/pregnant-eat-for-two-right.

Johnson, Melinda. "Is It Safe to Eat Sushi While Pregnant?" BabyCenter. July 2013. babycentre.co.uk/x568586/is-it-safe-to-eat -sushi-in-pregnancy.

Murkoff and Mazel. *What to Expect When You're Expecting*, 116, 117, 155, 156.

"What to Eat During Pregnancy." Medical News Today. July 15, 2013. medicalnewstoday.com/articles/246404.php.

Whitcomb, Lindsay L. "Is It Safe to Eat Deli Meats When I'm Pregnant?" BabyCenter. babycenter.com/406_is-it-safe-to-eat-deli-meats-when-im-pregnant_1246923.bc.

CRAVINGS AND SYMPATHY (WEIGHT) FOR THE DEVIL

Belkin, Lisa. "Men Gain Weight During Pregnancy." *New York Times.* June 2, 2009. parenting.blogs.nytimes.com/2009/06/02/men-who-swell-with-pregnancy/?_r=0.

Charlish and Davies. *The Complete Book of Natural Pregnancy and Childcare*, 29, 82, 89.

"Coping with Pregnancy Food Cravings." WebMD. June 1, 2006. webmd.com/baby/features/coping-with-pregnancy-food-cravings.

"Emotional Eating: Dealing with Cravings." Epigee: Women's Health. epigee.org/fitness/cravings.html.

Feld, Gina Bevinetto. "New Dads Gain Weight, Too." *American Baby.* June 2004. parents.com/parenting/dads/issues-trends/new-dads-gain-weight-too.

Murkoff and Mazel. *What to Expect When You're Expecting*, 155, 156.

O'Callaghan, Kitty. "Girl Talk: Sympathy Weight." Parenting.com. parenting.com/article/girl-talk-sympathy-weight.

"Pregnancy Food Cravings: What Pregnant Women Crave and Why." Epigee: Women's Health. epigee.org/pregnant_diet.html.

Taffinder, Darren. "The Perils of Pregnancy Sympathy-Weight." WeightWatchers. weightwatchers.com/util/art/index_art.aspx?tabnum=1&art_id=48241&sc=3053.

FOOD TIPS AND CALORIES

"The Pregnancy Diet: Protein." What to Expect. whattoexpect.com/pregnancy/eating-well/pregnancy-diet/protein.aspx.

"Seven Principles of Eating Well During Pregnancy." BabyCenter. babycenter.com/pregnancy-eating-well.

GO WITH THE FLOW

Charlish and Davies. *The Complete Book of Natural Pregnancy and Childcare*, 82, 89, 111, 120, 155, 248.

"Frequent Urination During Pregnancy." BabyCenter. babycenter .com/0_frequent-urination-during-pregnancy_237.bc.

"Melasma." National Institutes of Health. November 20, 2012. nlm .nih.gov/medlineplus/ency/article/000836.htm.

Murkoff and Mazel. *What to Expect When You're Expecting*, 15, 135, 342, 343.

Schwarz, Richard H. "Pregnancy and Urination." *American Baby*. parents.com/pregnancy/my-body/aches-pains/pregnancy -urination.

TIPS ON BRAXTON HICKS

"Braxton Hicks Contractions." American Pregnancy Association. October 2011. americanpregnancy.org/labornbirth/ braxtonhicks.html.

"Braxton Hicks Contractions." BabyCenter. babycenter.com/ 0_braxton-hicks-contractions_156.bc.

"Braxton-Hicks Contractions (False Labor)." MedicineNet. May 30, 2013. medicinenet.com/braxton_hicks_contractions/ article.htm.

"Labor and Delivery, Postpartum Care." Mayo Clinic. March 19, 2011. mayoclinic.org/healthy-living/labor-and-delivery/basics/ labor-and-delivery/hlv-20049465.

Murkoff and Mazel. *What to Expect When You're Expecting*, 311, 312, 359, 360.

Roizen and Oz. *YOU: Having a Baby*, 212, 227.

"Third Trimester Pregnancy: What to Expect." Mayo Clinic. December 4, 2012. mayoclinic.org/pregnancy/ART-20046767.

THE AMNIOCENTESIS TEST

"Amniocentesis." American Pregnancy Association. April 2006.
americanpregnancy.org/prenataltesting/amniocentesis.html.

"Amniocentesis." BabyCenter. August 2012. babycenter.com/
0_amniocentesis_327.bc.

Charlish and Davies. *The Complete Book of Natural Pregnancy and
Childcare*, 65, 139, 140, 143.

Murkoff and Mazel. *What to Expect When You're Expecting*, 64, 65.

"Pregnancy and Amniocentesis." WebMD. July 9, 2012. webmd
.com/baby/guide/amniocentesis.

DID YOU KNOW?

"Fetal Development: The Second Trimester." Mayo Clinic. December
4, 2012. mayoclinic.org/fetal-development/art-20046151.

"21 Amazing Facts About Your Pregnant Body." Babyexpert.com.
July 25, 2006. babyexpert.com/pregnancy/second-trimester/
21-amazing-facts-about-your-pregnant-body/1037.html.

. . . AND THEN THERE'S BOOBS/BOOBS: MYTHS VS. FACTS

"Breast Changes During Pregnancy." BabyCenter. babycenter
.com/0_breast-changes-during-pregnancy_262.bc.

Charlish and Davies. *The Complete Book of Natural Pregnancy and
Childcare*, 163, 263.

Murkoff and Mazel. *What to Expect When You're Expecting*, 335, 429,
441, 442.

Roizen and Oz. *YOU: Having a Baby*, 176–179, 252, 271.

Weiss, Robin Elise. "Myths About How Pregnancy and Breastfeeding Changes Your Breasts." About.com. pregnancy.about.com/
cs/breastfeeding1/a/aaaboutbreasts.htm.

GETTING CONNECTED WITH BABY

McCarthy, Laura Flynn. "What Babies Learn in the Womb." Parenting
.com. parenting.com/article/what-babies-learn-in-the-womb.

Roberts, Michelle. "Babies Can Hear Syllables in the Womb, Says Research." BBC News. February 25, 2013. bbc.co.uk/news/health-21572520.

Sanders, April. "When Can a Baby Hear in the Womb?" Modern-Mom. motherhood.modernmom.com/can-baby-hear-womb-11701.html.

"Unborn Babies Played Music in the Womb 'Remember the Melodies When They Are Born.'" *The Daily Mail*. March 8, 2011. dailymail.co.uk/sciencetech/article-1364120/Unborn-babies-played-music-womb-remember-melodies-born.html.

CHAPTER 3: THIRD TRIMESTER

"Fetal Development." American Pregnancy Association. January 2013. americanpregnancy.org/duringpregnancy/fetaldevelopment3.htm.

"Fetal Development: The Third Trimester." Mayo Clinic. December 4, 2012. mayoclinic.org/health/fetal-development/PR00114.

Murkoff and Mazel. *What to Expect When You're Expecting*, 328, 329, 342, 343.

Roizen and Oz. *YOU: Having a Baby*, 296, 297, 302, 303.

"Third Trimester of Pregnancy." What to Expect. whattoexpect.com/third-trimester-of-pregnancy.aspx.

"Third Trimester Symptoms." Parenting.com. parenting.com/article/third-trimester-symptoms.

DID YOU KNOW?

Doubilet, Peter, and Carol Benson. "Third Trimester Infant Development." Just the Facts, Baby. December 22, 2009. justthefactsbaby.com/pregnancy/article/third-trimester-infant-development-57.

"The Third Trimester." Johns Hopkins University. hopkinsmedicine
.org/healthlibrary/conditions/pregnancy_and_childbirth/
the_third_trimester_85,P01242.

MAKIN' DINNER FOR MOM

Jarosh, Willow, and Stephanie Clark. "A Week of Delicious Pregnancy Meals and Snacks." *Parents.* parents.com/pregnancy/
my-body/nutrition/prenatal-meal-plan.

"Germs: Understand and Protect Against Bacteria, Viruses and Infection." Mayo Clinic. April 30, 2011. mayoclinic.org/health/
germs/ID00002.

"Pregnancy Nutrition: Foods to Avoid During Pregnancy." Mayo Clinic. May 28, 2011. mayoclinic.org/health/pregnancy
-nutrition/ART-20043844.

GET YER ASS IN CLASS!

Roizen and Oz. *YOU: Having a Baby,* 155, 185, 190, 191, 296, 373.

THE HEAD SNAP

"Afraid of Breaking Baby." What to Expect. whattoexpect.com/
first-year/ask-heidi/afraid-of-breaking-baby.aspx.

"Caring for Your Baby." Pennsylvania Department of Health. www
.portal.state.pa.us/portal/server.pt/community/infant___new
born's_health/14173/caring_for_your_baby/558113.

CHOOSING THE BIRTHING PLACE

Charlish and Davies. *The Complete Book of Natural Pregnancy and Childcare,* 46, 180, 193, 439.

Dr. Kinch. "When to Go to the Emergency Room." BabyCenter. May 2, 2012. community.babycenter.com/post/a33064873/
when_to_go_to_the_emergency_room.

Roizen and Oz. *YOU: Having a Baby,* 227, 228, 233, 248, 249, 250, 297, 307, 336–338.

IN VITRO

"Infertility." American Pregnancy Association. May 2007. amer
icanpregnancy.org/infertility/ivf.html.

"In Vitro Fertilization (IVF): Definition." Mayo Clinic. June 27,
2013. mayoclinic.org/health/in-vitro-fertilization/MY01648.

THE NAME GAME

Roizen and Oz. *YOU: Having a Baby*, 297.

CHAPTER 4: BIRTH

YOUR ROLE DURING LABOR/THE BABY'S HERE

"Apgar." National Institutes of Health. December 2, 2011. nlm.nih
.gov/medlineplus/ency/article/003402.htm.

Charlish and Davies. *The Complete Book of Natural Pregnancy and
Childcare*, 46, 178–180, 193, 362, 372, 439.

Eden, Elizabeth. "How to Prepare For Childbirth." Discovery: Fit &
Health. health.howstuffworks.com/pregnancy-and-parenting/
pregnancy/labor-delivery/how-to-prepare-for-childbirth.htm.

"Epidural Anesthesia." American Pregnancy Association. August
2007. americanpregnancy.org/labornbirth/epidural.html.

Lack, Evonne. "10 Smart Ways to Prepare for Your Baby's Birth."
BabyCenter. babycenter.com/0_10-smart-ways-to-prepare-for
-your-babys-birth_10328975.bc.

"Labor and Delivery: Preparing." What to Expect. whattoexpect
.com/pregnancy/labor-and-delivery/preparing.aspx.

Moyer, Melinda Wenner. "The Truth About Epidurals." *Slate*. January 11, 2012. slate.com/articles/health_and_science/medical_
examiner/2012/01/the_truth_about_epidurals.html.

Murkoff and Mazel. *What to Expect When You're Expecting*, 347, 353,
354, 355, 380–399.

"Preparing for Birth." BabyCenter. babycenter.com/childbirth
-planning-and-preparing.

Roizen and Oz. *YOU: Having a Baby*, 306.

DID YOU KNOW?

"Fetal Development: The Third Trimester." Mayo Clinic. December 4, 2012. mayoclinic.org/health/fetal-development/ART-20045997.

"Your Pregnancy: 37 Weeks." BabyCenter. babycenter.com/6_your-pregnancy-37-weeks_1126.bc.

MISCELLANEOUS BIRTH FACTS

Charlish and Davies. *The Complete Book of Natural Pregnancy and Childcare*, 260.

"Meconium Aspiration." KidsHealth. October 2011. kidshealth.org/parent/medical/lungs/meconium.html.

"Meconium Aspiration Syndrome." Johns Hopkins Children's Center. hopkinschildrens.org/meconium-aspiration-syndrome.aspx.

"Meconium: Possible Causes for Meconium in the Fluid." Birth.com.au. December 1, 2012. birth.com.au/Variations-of-the-3rd-and-4th-stages-of-labour/Meconium-possible-causes-for-meconium-in-the-fluid.

Murkoff and Mazel. *What to Expect When You're Expecting*, 302, 360, 364, 369, 397, 399, 422, 565.

"Pitocin." RXList.com. March 22, 2013. rxlist.com/pitocin-side-effects-drug-center.htm.

Weiss, Robin Elise. "Meconium." About.com. pregnancy.about.com/od/laborcomplications/a/meconium.htm.

POSTPARTUM BLEEDING

"Lochia: Postpartum Bleeding." What to Expect. whattoexpect.com/first-year/month-by-month/your-body-postpartum-week1.aspx.

Murkoff and Mazel. *What to Expect When You're Expecting*, 421, 422.

Murry, Mary M. "Postpartum Bleeding: How Much Is Too Much?"

Mayo Clinic. February 4, 2010. mayoclinic.org/health/postpartum-bleeding/MY01179.

"Persistent Postpartum Bleeding." *Baylor University Medical Center Proceedings* 13, no. 2 (April 2000): 183–186. ncbi.nlm.nih.gov/pmc/articles/PMC1312304.

"Bleeding After the Birth (Lochia)" BabyCenter. April 2013. babycentre.co.uk/a553465/bleeding-after-the-birth-lochia.

THE ABCS OF C-SECTIONS

Charlish and Davies. *The Complete Book of Natural Pregnancy and Childcare*, 137, 190, 200, 204, 243.

Murkoff and Mazel. *What to Expect When You're Expecting*, 320–324, 398, 399, 432, 433.

Sears, William, Martha Sears, Robert Sears, and James Sears. *The Baby Book: Everything You Need to Know About Your Baby from Birth to Age Two* (New York: Little, Brown & Company, 1993), 44, 45.

TO CUT OR NOT TO CUT

"Circumcision." KidsHealth. March 2013. kidshealth.org/parent/system/surgical/circumcision.html.

"Circumcision (Male): Definition." Mayo Clinic. September 5, 2012. mayoclinic.org/health/circumcision/MY01023.

"Complications of Circumcision." Stanford School of Medicine. newborns.stanford.edu/CircComplications.html.

"Explaining Claims of Medical Benefits." Circumcision Resource Center. circumcision.org/benefits.htm.

Krill, Aaron J., Lane S. Palmer, and Jeffrey S. Palmer. "Complications of Circumcision." *The Scientific World Journal* 11 (2011): 2458–2468. ncbi.nlm.nih.gov/pmc/articles/PMC3253617.

Neroulias, Nicole. "New California Law Prohibits Circumcision Bans." *USA Today*. October 3, 2011. usatoday30.usatoday

.com/news/religion/story/2011-10-03/circumcision-ban
-california/50647014/1.

Roizen and Oz. *YOU: Having a Baby,* 55, 233, 236, 238, 244, 245, 269.

Shapiro, Ellen. "American Academy of Pediatrics Policy State-
ments on Circumcision and Urinary Tract Infection." *Reviews
in Urology* 1, no. 3 (1999): 154–159. ncbi.nlm.nih.gov/pmc/
articles/PMC1477524.

BABY PARANOIA

"Child Passenger Safety." AAA/CAA Digest of Motor Laws. driv
inglaws.aaa.com/laws/child-passenger-safety.

Shakespeare, William, *The Taming of the Shrew* (Katharina, Act V,
scene ii).

Singh, Gurcharan, and G. Archana. "Unraveling the Mystery of
Vernix Caseosa." *Indian Journal of Dermatology* 53, no. 2.(2008):
54–60. ncbi.nlm.nih.gov/pmc/articles/PMC2763724.

"Vernix Caseosa." Dictionary.com. dictionary.reference.com/
browse/vernix+caseosa.

"Vernix Caseosa." Merriam-Webster. m-w.com/medical/vernix%20
caseosa.

"What Is Vernix Caseosa?" ParentWeb. parentweb.com/pregnancy/
your-babys-development/vernix-caseosa.php.

BURRITO TIME!

Charlish and Davies. *The Complete Book of Natural Pregnancy and
Childcare,* 285.

"Infant Sleep Facts." Heartswaddle.com. heartswaddle.com/infant
-sleep-facts.

Roizen and Oz. *YOU: Having a Baby,* 128, 130, 131.

"Swaddling: Is It Safe?" American Academy of Pediatrics. January
2, 2014. healthychildren.org/English/ages-stages/baby/diapers
-clothing/pages/Swaddling-Is-it-Safe.aspx.

"Swaddling Your Baby." BabyCenter. May 2013. babycenter.com/
0_swaddling-your-baby_125.bc.

"Why Swaddle?" Heartswaddle.com. heartswaddle.com/why
-swaddle.

CHAPTER 5: LIFE WITH BABY

BRINGING HOME BABY

Bonyata, Kelly. "Breastfeeding Your Newborn: What to Expect in
the Early Weeks." Kellymom.com. September 2, 2011. kellymom
.com/bf/normal/newborn-nursing.

Krieger, Liz. "First 24 Hours at Home with Your Baby." BabyCenter.
babycenter.com/0_first-24-hours-at-home-with-your
-baby_10345806.bc.

"Postpartum Depression." KidsHealth. July 2013. kidshealth.org/
parent/emotions/feelings/ppd.html.

"Postpartum Depression and Anxiety." BabyCenter. babycenter
.com/0_postpartum-depression-and-anxiety_227.bc.

"Postpartum Depression Definition." Mayo Clinic. September 11,
2012. mayoclinic.org/health/postpartum-depression/DS00546.

"Safety Restraints." Department of Motor Vehicles, New York State.
dmv.ny.gov/occupant.htm.

BREAST MILK

"Breast Milk Storage: Do's and Don'ts." Mayo Clinic. April 6, 2012.
mayoclinic.org/health/breast-milk-storage/MY00926.

Charlish and Davies. *The Complete Book of Natural Pregnancy and
Childcare*, 261–263, 267.

"Collection and Storage of Breastmilk." Medela. medelabreast
feedingus.com/tips-and-solutions/11/collection-and-storage
-of-breastmilk.

Murkoff and Mazel. *What to Expect When You're Expecting*, 429, 430,
442–444.

"Safely Storing Breast Milk." KidsHealth. January 2012. kidshealth
.org/parent/growth/feeding/breastfeed_storing.html.

FORMULA FACTS

"Bottle-Feeding Basics." BabyCenter. November 2013. babycentre
.co.uk/a752/bottle-feeding-basics.

"Breastfeeding vs. Formula Feeding." KidsHealth. January 2012.
kidshealth.org/parent/growth/feeding/breast_bottle_feeding
.html.

Charlish and Davies. *The Complete Book of Natural Pregnancy and
Childcare*, 272, 273.

"Feeding Your 1- to 3-Month-Old." KidsHealth. September 2011.
kidshealth.org/parent/growth/feeding/feed13m.html.

"Formula Feeding." BabyCenter. babycenter.com/baby-formula
-feeding.

"How Much and How Often." KidsHealth. January 2012. kidshealth
.org/parent/pregnancy_newborn/formulafeed/formulafeed
_often.html.

Roizen and Oz. *YOU: Having a Baby*, 120, 128, 260, 266, 271.

BABY-PROOFING

"Babyproofing." *Parents*. parents.com/baby/safety/babyproofing.

Roizen and Oz. *YOU: Having a Baby*, 185, 296.

4 WAYS TO PROTECT YOUR BABY

Roizen and Oz. *YOU: Having a Baby*, 185, 296.

Sager, Jeanne. "How to Handle Head Injuries." *Parents*. November
2010. parents.com/toddlers-preschoolers/injuries/first-aid/
how-to-handle-head-injuries.

Zhang, Sarah. "Is There Lead in Your House?" *Mother Jones*. January
2013. motherjones.com/environment/2013/01/lead-poisoning
-house-pipes-soil-paint.

THE WONDERFUL WORLD OF PETS

Geller, David. "Should I Keep My Pet Away from My Newborn?" BabyCenter. babycenter.com/404_should-i-keep-my-pet-away -from-my-newborn_9944.bc.

Gipps, Nikole. "How Do I Prepare My Pet for Our New Baby?" BabyCenter. babycenter.com/preparing-pets-for-babies.

"Introducing Your Pet and New Baby." Humane Society of the United Sates. July 24, 2012. humanesociety.org/animals/ resources/tips/pets_babies.html.

Millan, Cesar. "Introduce Your Dog to Your Baby." Cesar's Way. August 29, 2013. cesarsway.com/tips/yournewdog/introduce -your-dog-to-your-baby.

Murkoff and Mazel. *What to Expect When You're Expecting*, 292.

"Pet Meets Baby." Humane Society of the United States. american humane.org/assets/pdfs/animals/pet-meets-babypdf.pdf.

Roizen and Oz. *YOU: Having a Baby*, 58, 274, 276, 295, 297

"Toxoplasmosis." KidsHealth. September 2011. kidshealth.org/ parent/infections/parasitic/toxoplasmosis.html.

"Toxoplasmosis: Definition." Mayo Clinic. June 24, 2011. mayoclinic .org/health/toxoplasmosis/DS00510.

"Toxoplasmosis During Pregnancy." BabyCenter. August 2012. babycenter.com/0_toxoplasmosis-during-pregnancy_1461.bc.

SEX AFTER BIRTH

Jio, Sarah. "The Truth About Sex After Pregnancy." *Woman's Day*. womansday.com/sex-relationships/sex-tips/the-truth-about-sex -after-pregnancy-91928.

"Kegel Exercises: Treating Male Urinary Incontinence." WebMD. June 12, 2012. webmd.com/urinary-incontinence-oab/kegel -exercises-treating-male-urinary-incontinence.

"Let's Talk About Sex: After the Baby." BabyCenter. babycenter .com/0_lets-talk-about-sex-after-the-baby_11802.bc.

Roizen and Oz. *YOU: Having a Baby,* 174.

"Sex After Pregnancy: Set Your Own Timeline." Mayo Clinic. July
    10, 2012. mayoclinic.org/health/sex-after-pregnancy/PR00146.

"Urinary Incontinence: Pelvic Organ Prolapse." WebMD. Ovtober
    7, 2010. webmd.com/urinary-incontinence-oab/tc/pelvic
    -organ-prolapse-topic-overview.

Woods, Stacey Grenrock. "How Different Is Sex Going to Be After
    My Wife Has Our Baby?" *Esquire.* August 2013. esquire.com/
    women/sex/sex-after-baby-0913.

MAN VS. MYTH

Linton, Bruce. "The Five Myths of Fatherhood." Fathers' Forum
    Online. fathersforum.com/articles?id=22.

Additional Reading
and Other Good Stuff

HELPFUL PARENTING WEBSITES AND BLOGS

Babble.com—A one-stop shop for all the information you need pertaining to parenting, travel, beauty, home, and entertainment.

Babycenter.com—Expert advice from around the globe on pregnancy, children's health, parenting, and more.

Whattoexpect.com—A terrific online resource that tracks your pregnancy from week to week and connects you with other parents to chat in open forums about pregnancy, parenting, and child-related topics.

Redtri.com—A sweet place to find cool ideas for things to do, eat, see, and make with your kids.

Parents.com—Expert advice about pregnancy, your life, and family time from the editors of *Parents* magazine.

Parenting.com—From recipes, mom-tested gear recommendations, photo galleries, and mom tips, *Parenting* magazine's one-stop online resource is the place for moms and moms-to-be.

GOOD READS

What to Expect When You're Expecting by Heidi Murkoff and Sharon Mazel (Workman Publishing Company)

Belly Laughs: The Naked Truth About Pregnancy and Childbirth by Jenny McCarthy (Da Capo Press)

The Girlfriends' Guide to Pregnancy by Vicki Iovine (Pocket Books)

The Happiest Baby on the Block by Harvey Karp (Bantam)

5 MUST-HAVES FOR YOUR NEWBORN

When it comes to baby gear there are plenty of choices on the market. Here are five items I feel you need to definitely include on your list:

- **Honest Company products:** Honest.com is our trusted source for stylish, eco-friendly, natural diapers, organic wipes, organic bath and body care, and nontoxic cleaning products. Honest .com.

- **Diaper Dude bag:** I know I may not be objective about this one, but you definitely need to get yourself a Diaper Dude bag. Choices range from our traditional black or camouflage to eco-friendly fabrics and licensed Major League Baseball–themed designs. There is a style for everyone at diaperdude .com.

- **Arm & Hammer Diaper Pail by Munchkin:** Powered by natural, odor-eliminating baking soda, the Arm & Hammer Diaper Pail helps keep your baby's nursery smelling fresh and clean. Munchkin.com.

- **Puj Tub:** The Puj Tub is the easiest baby bathtub ever. Made from a soft foam that folds and conforms to almost any sink, the Puj Tub cradles and protects the baby during bathtime. Pujbaby.com.

- **Baby carrier:** What better way to bond with your little one than by contact? Having a carrier you can trust to hold your precious cargo goes without saying. Check out Boba carriers (bobafamily .com) for a style that is both fashionable and safe.

Acknowledgments

One of the most interesting moments I spent with my wife when we were first dating was at her therapist's office. She had brought me along to discuss how serious I was about her. Talk about balls. She was lucky I didn't run away right then and there. Fortunately, I discovered a world I never wanted to leave. Hell, I was the fifth of six kids. I never got to get a word in edgewise growing up, so having someone who actually wanted me to talk was a dream. Needless to say, over sixteen years later, I am still committed to my personal growth and am still passionate about therapy. With that said, I have graced the chairs of many a therapist in New York and LA. They have been tremendous in being a guide to getting me where I am today. So to Barbara, Cecile, Sherry, Betsy, Josie, Mark, Susan, Don, Roberta, and Ruth I give you my heartfelt thanks. I know my work is not yet done so don't fret.

Thanks also to Akiko, my right-hand confidant at Diaper Dude headquarters. Without your talent and dedication, this book would've been impossible to complete.

Elana, Jeff, and the whole Rose Group family—thanks for being my champion in the early years. You saw a vision, and without your guidance I would have just been another dude on the block.

To Shab, Robert, Katie, Danielle, Hilary, Nichole, and Alecia at Flutie Entertainment—thanks for your belief in me. You are a dream team and made my dream a reality.

Stacey Glick, I feel honored to be working with you and your team. Thanks for the opportunity and being so amazing at your work.

Meg, I knew the moment we all had our first conference call that this book was meant to be with you and your team. I was thrilled you got my "voice" and didn't think I was some crazy, wacked-out dude. It has been an amazing experience working with you, and I am forever thankful to have had this opportunity.

Scott, thank you for taking the time and energy to share your input. You were a tremendous support with your honesty and constructive criticism. I knew you'd be the go-to guy when I needed to really hear the truth. Next night out is on me.

Danny, thanks for your honesty when being interviewed by your boss. You are always a pleasure to see each day at work. Thanks for your dedication.

A special thanks to Dr. Holly Lucille for your guidance and expertise on the book.

Frank, my other voice—dude, to say this book would not have been possible without you is an understatement. You challenged me when I needed to up my game and made me a better writer for it. Thanks for all your hard work and dedication. This experience felt the furthest from work because of your talent.

To my wife, Meredith, I say thank you for letting me put our experience out there for others to learn and grow by. You are such an amazing partner, friend, mother, teacher, and proofreader. If not for you, this book would never have been possible. Thanks for reading and rereading, editing and suggesting over and over again. Your passion is such an inspiration. Without your belief in me, I would have given up at the moment this book entered my mind. I love you!

Finally this book would never have been possible without my children.

Kai, Juliette, and Cole, you have all truly been a gift that has brought so much love and happiness to my life. I love you guys.

. . . *plus* . . .

Frank Meyer would like to extend his heartfelt thanks to Shab Azma, Stacey Glick, Meg Leder, and Djiji. Without your help, this book would not have been possible.

Chris, thank you for the opportunity to help you tell your story. We make a great team and it has been a pleasure.

And thank you to the light of my life, my daughter, Bella. You make me who I am today.

Index

About the Authors

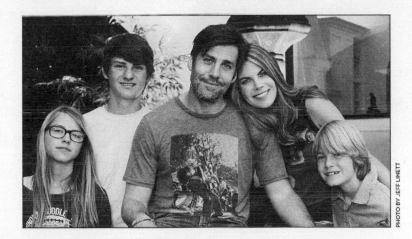

Actor-turned-father-turned-designer **Chris Pegula** is the creator of Diaper Dude, America's most high-profile line of hip gear for cool dads. After the birth of the first of his three children, Pegula noticed that most diaper bags and accessories were designed with women's sense of style in mind and created the Diaper Dude for dads. In addressing a simple need, Pegula revolutionized an industry. He has since been featured on *Rachael Ray, Ellen, The Nate Berkus Show, E! News*, HGTV's *Gotta Have It!, The Oprah Winfrey Show*, and numerous other TV and radio spots. Since the launch of Diaper Dude, Chris has emerged as a lifestyle expert on all things family-, parenting-, and partner-related. The Diaper Dude is not just a bag . . . it's a way of life. *From Dude to Dad: The Diaper Dude Guide to Pregnancy* is the first step in how to achieve that way of life.

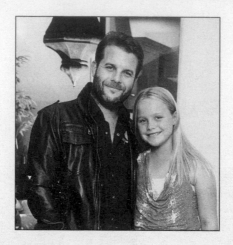

Telly- and Webby-award-winning author **Frank Meyer** is senior content producer at NBC's Esquire Network. He penned *When the Wall of Sound Met the New York Underground: The Ramones, Phil Spector and End of the Century* and is coauthor of *On the Road with the Ramones* (so clearly he likes the Ramones!). Frank has written features for *Variety, Yahoo!, LA Weekly,* and *New Times,* edited Neil Zlozower's *Van Halen: A Visual History,* and is the front man of punk band the Streetwalkin' Cheetahs. Frank is also the proud single father of a ten-year-old girl, who loves soccer and reading. Her first concert with her dad was KISS!